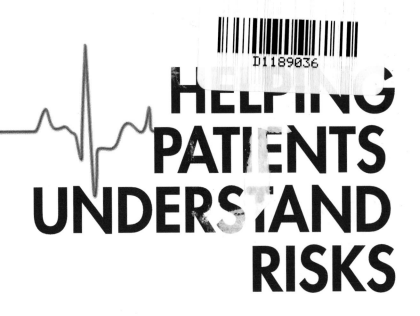

HELPING
PATIENTS
UNDERSTAND
RISKS

7

Simple Strategies
For Successful Communication

John Paling PhD

The Risk Communication Institute

Helping Patients Understand Risks
Seven simple strategies for successful communication.

Published by: The Risk Communication Institute,
5822 NW 91 Boulevard, Gainesville, Florida 32653-2864

ISBN-10: 0-9642236-7-8
ISBN-13: 978-0-9642236-7-7

1.Title 2. Visual Aids for Risk Communication 3.Healthcare Communication 4. Improving Doctor-Patient Partnerships 5. Decision Aids.

For information contact:
The Risk Communication Institute,
5822 NW 91 Boulevard, Gainesville, Florida 32653-2864
(352) 377-2142   www.riskcomm.com

This book is dedicated to:

All health professionals who want to be more effective at helping patients understand their risks

All hospitals that seek to provide patient–focused communications

All pharmaceutical companies and regulatory agencies that want the general public to understand the true facts about medical products and services

Warning — Disclaimer

This book is designed to provide general information about how healthcare professionals might more effectively communicate to patients about risks. It is sold with the understanding that the publisher and author are not medically qualified and that none of the material in this book is intended to serve as guidance for the reader's personal decisions with regard to acceptable risks, appropriate procedures or medical alternatives. People seeking authoritative information about their own concerns should consult with their own medical professionals.

While every effort has been made to make this book as accurate as possible, there may be mistakes both typographical and in content. Thus, this text should be used only as a general guide and not as the ultimate source on this topic.

The purpose of this book is to educate and to entertain. The author and The Risk Communication Institute (and all groups or organizations with which the author is involved) shall have neither liability nor responsibility to any person or entity with respect to any loss or damage caused, or alleged to have been caused, directly or indirectly by the information contained in or omitted from this book.

If you do not wish to be bound by the above, you may return this book to the publisher for a full refund.

> *I truly believe that those doctors who are responsible for patients have the most difficult challenges in all of risk communication..* John Paling

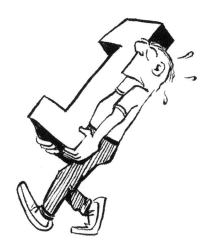

Being number one is a heavy burden to carry

About the Author

John Paling PhD was born in England and started his career as a junior professor in zoology at Oxford University. There, as well as doing research, he became a popular lecturer in the community and was impressed by the ability of visual media to communicate across all divisions of society. With four colleagues, he founded an international wildlife movie company which made the very first (American) PBS Nova television program that went on to win an Emmy Award. This lead to over two decades traveling the world filming, producing and presenting documentary films for television.

Paling moved to the USA in 1980 and, shortly afterwards, made a film on alligators for The National Geographic Society that was awarded two more Emmys. (This experience led to the title of his first book on risks *Up to your armpits in alligators?*)

Over this time he was also Regents Professor at the University of California, Santa Cruz and on the faculty in three different departments at the University of Florida. Additionally, for most of his adult life he has been in demand as a keynote speaker for international meetings. (His presentations are distinctive because he includes short segments from his wildlife films to serve as metaphors for his main messages.)

All these experiences finally led him into the world of risk communication when one of his clients, the Environmental Protection Agency, introduced him to the challenges of explaining risks to the public. The same problems were troubling many of his major corporate clients as they were frequently being challenged to explain the risks associated with their products and services to an increasingly concerned and skeptical public.

To answer this challenge, Paling designed a series of "Richter Scales for Risks" to show people a context for the different risks in life. His work led to a book that was featured by *Scientific American* and, as a result of that publicity, doctors started to contact him asking to use his communication tools in their work with patients.

He found himself coauthoring specialist papers on communicating risks to patients in a variety of peer-reviewed journals, and it dawned on him that his work could be useful in a whole range of different healthcare specialties. Having been adopted by the medical profession, Paling was surprised to find that many of the lessons for effective risk communication already used in other professions had never found their way into healthcare. He was also stunned to realize that many of the risks in the healthcare arena were far more likely, and far more serious, than those that he had been working on in other aspects of society. For this reason, as well as the special circumstances of the doctor-patient relationship, he went on to invent his "Paling Palette©," a different communication aid that is often better suited to the needs of doctors.

In 2003, the *British Medical Journal* commissioned Paling to write an article[1] about his "toolbox of ideas" for improving risk communication. After that, even more medical organizations have sought his services as they have come to recognize that simple improvements in this field can lead to significant benefits both for themselves and for their patients.

John is founder and research director for The Risk Communication Institute, a company providing speaking and consulting services to organizations worldwide.

John and his wife Wendy live on a small lake in North Florida. He still makes wildlife movies but now only as a hobby. His passion is to improve one small, but important, corner of healthcare by sharing his unique insights and materials that could only have come about as the culmination of his own professional journey.

> *We can't receive wisdom.*
> *We must discover it for ourselves*
> *after a journey that no one can take*
> *for us or spare us.*
>
> *Marcel Proust: (French novelist)*

Illustrated by Don Baumgart

For many years, Don Baumgart was a high school principal in Wisconsin where he is still active as a Town Supervisor in his local community. He has double masters degrees in fine arts and education and his cartoons have graced many different books and articles on a wide range of topics. He adds great pleasure to life for all who view his work. His personal warmth is invariably reflected in his gentle and empathetic humor.

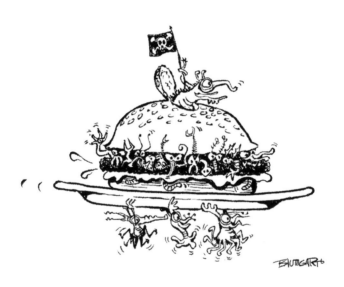

Sometimes risks get exaggerated in patients' minds

The Illustrations

In places, this book takes a flippant (some may think, inappropriate) approach to the serious topic of risk communication.

Please know that the illustrations and the occasional lighthearted text are intended as "the spoonful of sugar to help the medicine go down."

From the outset, I predicted that an ordinary book with this title would only appeal to the relatively few people who were already studying this field anyway. These experts were not my target audience.

Instead, my goal was to appeal to the widest possible range of health professionals in the hope that many more doctors would be introduced to and then embrace some of the simple improvements that are offered here. In other words, we tried to take account of how busy healthcare professionals are and, in response, we have purposely tried to produce an appealing book that is easy to digest.

However, humor is a personal thing and what appeals to some may not appeal to everyone. Indeed, like communication between doctors and patients, there can easily be misunderstandings that were never intended or expected.

In other words, please don't mistake our attempts to entertain you as you read with a lack of respect or empathy for all those who are suffering in any way. The reality of the risks that patients struggle to understand is of course no laughing matter.

How well we communicate is determined not by how well we say things but how well we are understood.

Andrew Grove, Co-founder of Intel

Table of Contents

Why This Book Was Written

There are three main reasons why this book was created:

- To introduce healthcare professionals to simple new visual aids to help them explain risks to their patients.

- To stimulate doctors to test these communications tools in their own fields and then to independently report on their effectiveness in improving patient understanding.

- To show that in the cost-conscious world of healthcare, there are still many opportunities to improve patient care in ways that take effectively no extra time or money.

FOREWORD

The reader will see immediately that this is not like other books for health professionals. Instead of being uniformly scholarly in tone and appearance, it reflects the personalities of the author and illustrator who happen to come from different professions yet bring unique expertise and credentials to the mission of this book. To avoid any misunderstandings, let us make clear what this work is – and isn't.

What this book is

This book provides a "toolbox of strategies" – including specially designed decision aids – for all those who want to be more effective at communicating risks with patients. It highlights research studies that show where patients have problems understanding risks and then offers simple solutions that we believe are significant improvements on the current practices in the profession. Once readers become aware of the need for and the benefits of these tools, they are encouraged to try them out for themselves in their own special fields. On-going help and collaboration are offered for those who wish to feel better at effectively communicating the true facts about risks to patients and their families.

What this book isn't

This book is not a compendium of specific risks for different healthcare topics. Readers will already have far more knowledge and understanding of the risks and benefits associated with their specialty than the author.

It is also not intended as a review of medical decision-making nor, frankly, is it the solution to many of the complex choices that patients face in modern healthcare treatments.

And it is certainly not the last word on the topic. Rather the book is intended to parallel the author's seminars and conference presentations that encourage doctors who may never have studied risk communication before to apply the principles of patient-focused care.

WHERE TO START

Because doctors are so busy, this book offers five different prescriptions for treating doctors with different needs.

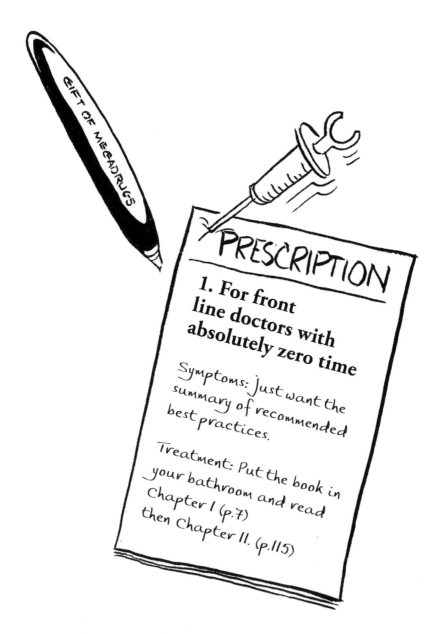

GIFT OF MEGADRUGS

PRESCRIPTION

1. For front line doctors with absolutely zero time

Symptoms: Just want the summary of recommended best practices.

Treatment: Put the book in your bathroom and read Chapter I (p.7) then Chapter II. (p.115)

PRESCRIPTION

2. For doctors just wanting solutions

Symptoms: Reader only wants the recommended strategies and the visual aids.

Treatment: Put the book in your pocket. Start at Chapter 1 (p.7) then skip to page 71 and read during coffee and lunch breaks.

PRESCRIPTION

3. For most readers

Symptoms: Reader wants to learn of the recommended strategies <u>after</u> understanding where patients encounter difficulties.

Treatment: Put the book by your bedside and read prior to sleep.

PRESCRIPTION

4. For more experienced, senior doctors

Symptoms: Readers feel that this book offers valuable tools that "someone" should test and report on.

Treatment: Delegate the task to junior doctors or residents. Start at page 161 for practical assistance for how to set up studies.

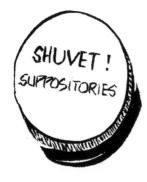

SHUVET!
SUPPOSITORIES

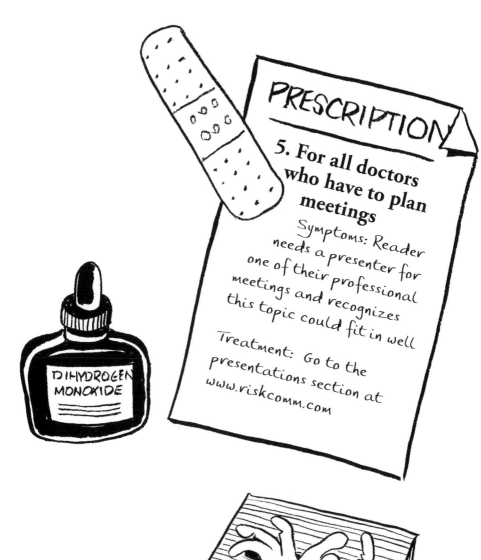

PRESCRIPTION

5. For all doctors who have to plan meetings

Symptoms: Reader needs a presenter for one of their professional meetings and recognizes this topic could fit in well

Treatment: Go to the presentations section at www.riskcomm.com

DIHYDROGEN MONOXIDE

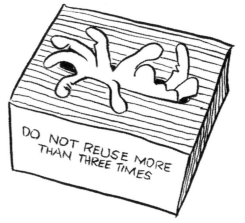

DO NOT REUSE MORE THAN THREE TIMES

Some Simplifications

This book primarily focuses on the communication challenges of physicians dealing with individual patients. However, many of the lessons that follow will also apply to public health officials and drug companies whose target audience is the population at large. Readers interested in public health issues should also review the compilation of papers in Bennett and Calman.[1]

For simplicity, I am going to use the words "doctors" or "physicians" as shorthand for all the other health professionals who can benefit from the strategies that follow.

Similarly, to avoid the need to constantly refer to both genders ("his or her" etc.), I have decided to speak of doctors as being male and genetic counselors and patients as being female. I reverted to this format after consciously trying to change the out-dated image in order to publicize the superior performance of the many women professionals in healthcare communications (see chapter 15). In fact, the first two drafts of this book were formulated in the reverse convention and it was women reviewers who suggested that I bow to the dominant numbers in each class and stop straining to be politically correct. Since then, however, other women doctors have bridled at my choice which they see as insensitive and reinforcing the stereotype.

All this makes me realize that, like other well-intentioned attempts to communicate effectively, you don't always get it right – and that emotions can dominate decisions and reactions, whatever the topic.

Finally, the reader should keep in mind that this book has been written primarily from the perspective of the healthcare system in the USA. Some of the ideas may need to be adapted or even rejected in other cultures.

However, having said that, I still spend a good deal of time in my original homeland of England and have spoken at many conferences internationally. These experiences lead me to believe that – immaterial of the differences of cultures – the visual communication tools and strategies described in this book can work in all countries.

THE SEVEN SIMPLE STRATEGIES FOR HELPING PATIENTS UNDERSTAND RISKS

1 Prepare by first learning about the actual difficulties that patients experience in attempting to understand risks.

2 Accept the challenge that patients' emotions will invariably filter the facts and cannot be ignored.

3 Revise the way you explain probabilities to patients. The most commonly-used methods can be greatly improved with small changes.

4 Try to avoid speaking to patients in terms of relative risks. Ensure you provide context so patients get "information" and not just "data."

5 Never just give the negative perspective but, instead, make sure the positive perspective is always provided as well.

6 Explain the risk numbers by using visual aids. These give context as well as achieving understanding for the largest number of patients.

7 Realize that sharing visual aids with patients can serve to reinforce the doctor-patient bond, enhance trust and encourage acceptance of the doctor's message.

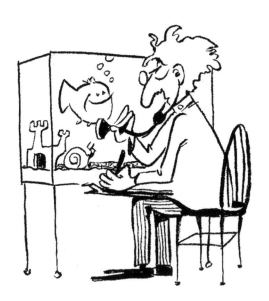

Don't ask a fish!

INTRODUCTION

If you want to know what water is, don't ask a fish!

I truly believe that those doctors who are responsible for patients have the most difficult challenges in all of risk communication.

I sincerely salute the profession and want to make clear at the outset that my motivation for writing this book was emphatically not to criticize. Rather I simply wanted to lay out a menu of new ideas that I strongly believe will make for more effective communication between doctors and patients. More specifically, I believe this book will improve patient understanding while also increasing the satisfaction that doctors get from doing their job. In short, adopting the strategies in these pages can make their days go better.

Let's begin by being honest with each other.

Many readers are likely to start this book with a healthy dose of skepticism. After all, they have been successfully doing informed consents for many years and they've never had to read a book to tell them how to do it!

These are natural responses so I simply invite anyone who starts off with this view to keep an open mind. My justification for writing this can be summarized by the maxim. "If you want to know what water is – don't ask the fish!"

Many doctors have been so immersed in the process for so long that they may never have had a chance to see it from the fresh perspective of those who have never swum in their particular sea. That's the mind-set that emboldens me, a strange fish from a different ocean, to offer doctors the essence of over ten years of teaching and research on effective risk communication in industries other than healthcare.

LESSONS FROM OTHER PROFESSIONS

If anyone still needs convincing about the value of a fresh approach, consider this: From the perspective of people who deal in risk communication in other disciplines, doctors are definitely the odd group out.

In every other industry where risks have to be communicated to the public (e.g. chemical, nuclear, food and water) there is widespread awareness that it is not an easy task and that there can be costly consequences when it is done poorly. As a result, there are usually only a very few spokespeople who do risk communication on behalf of their industries and they are all very highly trained.

In contrast, in healthcare (where incidentally, the risks are usually far greater and far more uncertain and complex) almost every clinician in the world communicates risks to patients and virtually none of them have had any training for it whatsoever!

It is not formally taught in medical schools and although a few specialist groups such as The Society for Medical Decision Making do offer their members academic courses in the field[1], to the best of my knowledge, this is the only book that focuses on communicating risks to individual patients.

In fact, in my opinion risk communication in healthcare is still in the Dark Ages. Young doctors learn their skills like apprentices in a medieval guild. They just pick up what to do by watching the master craftsman. There is rarely any formal training or any awareness of how their profession is behind the times compared to others. Here is another striking fact that drives that point home:

All professional journalists and television producers who want to show the significance of numbers in the media are trained to use visual aids such as pie charts or graphs.

In contrast, in healthcare there has been no tradition for using visual aids to improve patient understanding of the risk numbers.

Significantly, one of the main ingredients of this book is to introduce visual aids into medical risk communication. This reinforces my belief that a fish from a different sea can bring real value to healthcare professionals.

It is always a temptation for doctors to fall back on the same mental approach that is comfortable and reflects how MDs think about risks within the profession. The challenge, of course, is for the clinician to communicate in the way that the patient is most likely to understand. To do this, it is imperative that the physician has insight into the patient's needs and perspective.

This book starts by outlining the many challenges to effectively communicating risks to patients and then moves on to suggest solutions.

The term "risk" appears in the title of more than 2% of all the medical articles published in 2004.

Elmore and Gigerenzer[2]

SECTION ONE

SUMMARY OF BEST PRACTICES

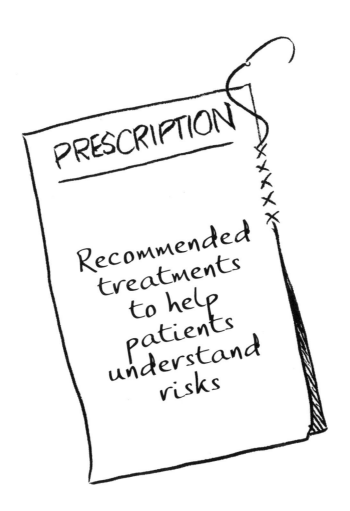

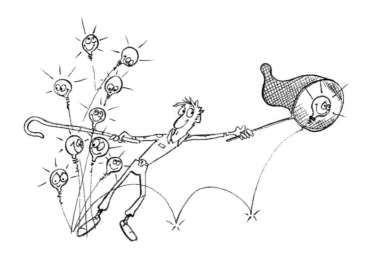

Bright Ideas Worth Capturing.

1

SEVEN STRATEGIES FOR SUCCESS

The whole essence of the book
within one short chapter..

The next few pages summarize the major strategies that we recommend. If busy doctors just followed these simple steps, I am sure that:

1. Patients would better understand their risks and choices, and
2. Doctors would feel better about how they carry out this challenging responsibility.

This "toolbox" of techniques for effective risk communication includes best practices that have been largely overlooked in healthcare yet are widely used by professionals who are trained to explain risks in other professions (chemical, nuclear, food and drink, etc.).

In addition, this book introduces innovative visual aids that have been designed to meet the special needs of doctors. These tools enable patients to "see" their risks in a meaningful context.

1. First learn the difficulties that patients actually experience.

It turns out that patients have far greater obstacles to understanding risks than limitations in their education.

Most physicians have been doing risk communication for years and, by and large, they feel that they do it perfectly well. Because biomedical matters are the prime focus of their training, they typically learn about explaining risks by watching their senior colleagues. This results in the profession still viewing risk communication as a largely intuitive skill that can be picked up by cultural osmosis.

However, in this closed cycle, success tends to be evaluated by the *feelings* of the doctor as opposed to the *understanding* of the patient. When viewed from a patient-focused perspective, we see that **the ways that most doctors explain risks to patients can be needlessly confusing, often provide data but not information and, unwittingly, can actually be harmful to the patients' best interests.**

The doctor's first task should be to become aware of the reasons why risk communication can be so difficult. Later they can embrace tools and strategies that will optimize patient understanding.

Most healthcare professionals come to a risk communication seminar with the prime goal of learning better ways to communicate the numbers. This book answers that need. However, it is clear that the patient's emotions and attitudes can dominate how the doctor's communication is received; a reality that also must be taken into account.

Table 1 shows some of the reasons why risk communication can be very difficult to do well.

> *Seek first to understand*
> *and then to be understood.*
>
> — *Stephen R. Covey*

Table 1: Challenges to effective risk communication

Many Patients

- Assess risks primarily on emotions rather than on facts.

- Consistently misunderstand which are the more likely risks when their doctor quotes numbers to explain the odds of different possibilities.

- Massively overreact to expressions of relative risks leaving them unduly influenced by the media, health agencies, and pharmaceutical companies.

- Differ very widely in their wishes for involvement.

- Don't have the necessary education to really understand the complexities of modern medicine.

- Are influenced more by social contacts, advertising and media reports than by the knowledge of their doctors.

Many Doctors

- Are so focused on evidence-based decision making that they see their main task as being better at communicating the key numbers to their patients.

- Are unaware that they can alter their patients' perceptions and decisions simply by whether they present the risk numbers from the positive or the negative perspective.

- Do not know that simple visual aids can show patients the key numbers in a meaningful context – including the positive as well as the negative perspective.

- Are uncertain about how much detail to provide to patients due to a concern that telling the full truth may not be in the patient's best interests.

- Have never been challenged to evaluate their methods of risk communication to see if they are only providing "data" and not "information."

- Have never been introduced to the lessons of effective risk communication from other professions.

Many Doctors & Patients

Use the same descriptive words (e.g. "low risk") while meaning entirely different things.

Many Healthcare Organizations

- View informed consent as much a risk management strategy for the institution as a source of useful information for the patient.

- Are content with the status quo, since it is legally defensible.

2. Accept what cannot be changed, namely . . .

Patients' emotions will invariably filter the facts and cannot be ignored.

Doctors often view patients' emotions as an obstacle to sound decision-making and wish instead that they would focus their attention on the facts. In response to this, **doctors come to hope that some way will be found to overcome the emotional barriers that patients erect.**

We now recognize that this is an unhelpful illusion. A patient's emotions are fundamental to how choices are made. It is basic human nature. This explains why in every generation, large sections of the public embrace unproven medical solutions based purely on their feelings of trust for the product, the practitioner, or an unqualified but convincing friend. It is easy to speculate on why humans are hard-wired to respond in this manner. From ancestral times, the many risks to their lives could only be evaluated in human or emotional terms.

In other words, it is futile for doctors to try to overcome or marginalize a patient's emotional responses to risk information. Instead physicians must accept that the sometimes derided "soft factors" will always influence the patient's understanding of and decisions about the risks of life. This does not mean pampering patients or avoiding the hard truths. **Doctors will be most effective at communicating the facts about risks when they consciously reinforce their patients' perceptions of competence and caring.**

This emotional filter also explains the dozen or so factors that routinely color people's perceptions about the risks of life – *irrespective of what the actual numbers tell us about what is really the most likely risk.* (See Table 2.)

> *Communication without compassion is brutality.*
>
> — *Sharon Johnson, IBM*

Table 2: Emotional factors that influence what the public sees as a big risk irrespective of what the statistics might indicate (These apply to all risks – not just medical risks.)

Category A: Who tells you

INCREASE IN FEAR - LARGE RISK

- Information comes from someone NOT showing both competence and caring for the patient = UNtrustworthy source

- Risk communicator is NOT unambiguously "on my side" – unresponsive or not clearly patient-focused

- Source is someone you don't know

DECREASE IN FEAR - SMALL RISK

- Information comes from someone showing both competence and caring for the patient = Trustworthy source

- Risk communicator IS unambiguously "on my side" – responsive, supportive and empathetic

- Source is family member or friend

Category B: What type of risk it is

INCREASE IN FEAR - LARGE RISK

- Involuntary or coerced – e.g. "I want you to take these..."

- Industrial or produced by industry

- Catastrophic – Many affected at one time

- Unfamiliar – something we are not used to, e.g. genetically modified foods

- Dreaded > other risks, e.g. cancer

- Exposure NOT controlled by you

- Memorable – Personal awareness of harm caused by the risk in question

- Unfair or immoral burden on certain people, e.g. poor folk more at risk

DECREASE IN FEAR - SMALL RISK

- Voluntary, freely chosen – not coerced e.g. "How about if we try these ...?

- Natural – e.g. health foods

- Chronic – e.g. car crashes vs plane crashes

- Familiar – been around for a long time, e.g. flu, anaesthesia

- Less dreaded, e.g. heart disease

- Exposure to the risk controlled by you

- Not particularly memorable

- "Just bad luck" – No one caused you to be more at risk than other people

3. Speak to your listener

Revise the way you explain probabilities and patient understanding will be improved.

Physicians should not expect that the common descriptive words they use to describe risks mean the same thing to patients. They probably won't! And the differences are not trivial. "Low risk" may mean a likelihood of 1 in 5 to some listeners and 1 in 10,000 to others. All the other descriptive words (rare, remote, high, moderate, possible, and qualifiers like "very", "rather", "quite," etc.) only have a clear meaning from the perspective of the person doing the communication – typically the doctor. Problems arise because patients use these same words themselves but often intending different levels of likelihood.

What is minor to a physician might not seem small to a patient. Table 3 offers a way of providing consistency.

At times, doctors may forget how educated they are compared to most patients. **For effective risk communication, then, doctors must communicate in language that takes into account how it will be "received" by the patient.** For instance, doctors are surprised to learn that over 40% of patients will confuse which probability is more likely to happen: 1 in 250 or 1 in 25.

By changing all the statements of odds into frequencies, it is unmistakable which option represents the bigger probability. (The above numbers would then transpose to 4 out of 1000 people as compared to 40 out of 1000 people.)

Notice that once translated into such a form, it is easier for folk of all educational levels (and language skills) to understand which is the greater. **This is a simple but important change that all doctors should try and embrace.**

> *Never mistake silence for agreement or understanding*
>
> *—Anon*

Table 3: A simple way to reduce misunderstanding over the use of descriptive terms

VERBAL CONSISTENCY

Several respected professionals across the world have suggested that physicians in the different medical specialties should draw up a *limited* vocabulary of descriptors that are consistently used and matched to different levels of probability. In that way, over time, patients will gain a more accurate understanding of what doctors really mean by their explanations.

Our suggested vocabulary of descriptive terms and odds is shown below. However, citizens of different countries might be more familiar with a slightly different sequence so adjustments should be made to take into account the country, language and culture. What is most important is that there is some clear meaning to the few descriptive terms used to describe probabilities.

Verbal Description	Odds
Very High	1 in 1 – 1 in 10
High	1 in 10 – 1 in 100
Moderate	1 in 100 – 1 in 1,000
Low	1 in 1,000 – 1 in 10,000
Very Low	1 in 10,000 – 1 in 100,000
Minimal	1 in 100,000 – 1 in 1 million
Effectively Zero	1 in 1 million – 1 in 1 billion

USE FREQUENCIES, NOT ODDS

Although many patients will continue to think in terms of "1 in —" numbers when they consider likelihoods, their familiarity with this common practice can actually be a hindrance when it comes to comparing different risks. A truly patient-focused doctor will look at the range of risks that he typically communicates to his patients and then *transpose the odds into frequencies with a common denominator* (usually how many out of 1000 people.)

For example, over a 5-year period, 15 out of 1000 post menopausal women are predicted to get breast cancer — even if they don't take hormone therapy. If they do take hormone therapy over that period, 19 out of 1000 can be expected to get the disease. It is immediately evident that this strategy for communicating likelihoods is far easier for patients to understand than comparing odds of 1 in 67 with the odds of 1 in 53. Frequencies immediately show we are dealing with a difference of 4 extra people out of 1000 over a 5-year period.

4. Don't use relative risks when you speak to patients.

They need to have a meaningful context before any communication can be considered "information."

Here are two important, interrelated strategies.

A. All healthcare organizations are committed to the concept of informing patients before they consent to treatment, yet many informed consent forms offer only data – not information. What's the difference? "Data" consists of bare facts: – a PSA reading of 8 or a cervical smear reading of II, or a likelihood of 1 in 400. In contrast, **true information is "facts presented in a meaningful context."** Effective risk communication requires that doctors try to communicate *an understandable context* as well as delivering the key facts.

B. For over a decade, experts in risk communication have been pointing out that statements of relative risks totally fail to provide "information" to patients because they have no context to know what, say, a "50% increased risk" is measured in relation to. In view of this universal condemnation of the practice, it is shameful when healthcare agencies, pharmaceutical companies and the media persist in making public pronouncements about risks or benefits solely in this manner. It is well known that if patients only hear data expressed as relative risks, they take away deceptively exaggerated impressions of the differences.

The patient-focused solution to this widespread practice is to provide the absolute numbers and make comparisons by using easy-to-understand visual aids.

Table 4 further explains how expressions of relative risk confuse and misinform the public.

Think like a wise man but communicate in the language of the people.

— William Butler Yeats

Table 4: Reasons to BAN relative risks from communications with the public

Relative risks can cause massive confusion for patients.

Here's an example.
Say that the records show that for a defined population of people, about 2 out of 100 are at risk of having a heart attack over the next year. Then imagine that a new study comes out reporting that if such patients take an aspirin daily, their risk of a heart attack will be lowered. Instead of 2 out of 100 suffering a heart attack, only 1 person out of 100 would be expected to do so.

You could hardly imagine a simpler risk communication scenario. Yet one doctor might tell the patient, "Aspirin reduces your risk of heart attack by 1%" while another doctor (using the same data) might say, "Aspirin reduces your risk by 50%."

The first doctor would be accurate in that he meant "the risk would normally be 2% but aspirin reduces those odds down to 1%." (This is a statement of absolute risk reduction.) But the second doctor would also be accurate and simply meant to communicate that, if you take aspirin, the risk is now halved; i.e. 50%; down from 2% to 1%. (This is a statement of relative risk.)

Relative risk statements always exaggerate the public's perception of the real effect.

50% feels far more dramatic than 1% which is why the media and sometimes drug companies encourage it. Yet Celebrex, Vioxx, Bextra and hormone replacement therapy drugs have all lost public confidence recently, in part because their risks were expressed in relative terms.

Conclusions:

1. For the public, relative risks represent miscommunication.
2. The healthcare profession should adopt policies to outlaw the practice of only using relative risks when talking to patients.

5. "Accentuate the positive . . ."

Never just give the negative perspective but instead make sure that the positive perspective is also provided.

If a patient hears about a possible treatment that comes with a 3% chance that she will die, then she will almost certainly turn down that option. On the other hand, if the same scenario is offered and the predicted outcome is explained as "There is a 97% chance that this will cure you," most patients will accept it. On hearing of any risk purely from the negative perspective, a patient's emotions will typically exaggerate the likelihood of the bad outcome.

Unarguably, the human mind can play an important role in the healing process, given positive expectations of the outcomes. Therefore, it is counterproductive when doctors frame risks *only* from the negative perspective, thus reducing the opportunity for hope and the potential benefits of the placebo effect to operate.

The best way to help patients is to make sure you also include the numbers of those who will not be affected or suffer. This is equally honest yet it generates a different attitude in the mind of the patient.

A communication tool that shows both perspectives

Doctors must stay alert to this issue of "framing" the information they present and ensure they **include the positive aspect of the treatment** while addressing their patients' concerns.

We now offer visual aids that make this simple for doctors to achieve – and for patients to understand. On one graphic, the doctor can show the estimated numbers who will *not* be affected, as well as those who might be. **See Figure 5**.

> *They are able because*
> *they think they are able.*
>
> *— Virgil*

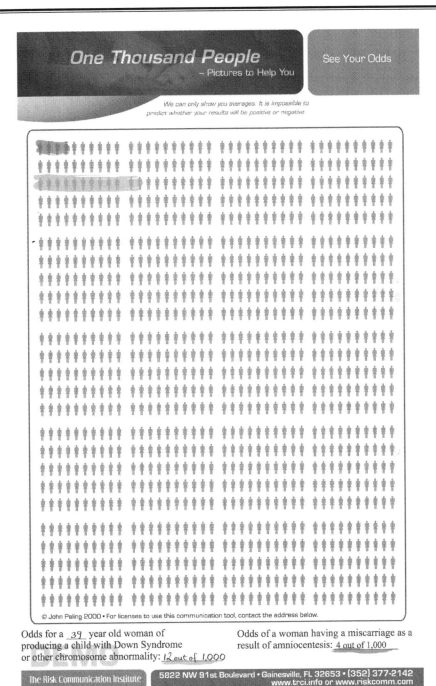

Figure 5: How to show those who are not likely to be affected – *as well as those who are*

6. Explain risk numbers by using visual aids.

These give context as well as helping the largest number of patients see what the doctor means.

A large part of risk information is always going to involve explaining the numbers data in some sort of context. We have designed two main styles of visual aids specifically for risk communication.

1. The Paling Palettes© (Figure 5). These are layouts of 1000 icons of little people which allow doctors to show the absolute (not the relative) number of people who may be affected – and those NOT likely to be harmed. These palettes are vividly simple and effective. They provide a good demonstration of the truth of the journalists' maxim, "One picture is worth a thousand words."

2. The Paling Perspective Scale©. This tool provides a consistent framework that can:

a. Display the odds of one risk and compare it to another. This should always be done cautiously, if possible "comparing apples with apples." (For important information on this tool, please refer to the corresponding section of the book.)

b. Address the "home-base" zone. This home-base zone is the place where the many risks that the general public is "at home with" fall on the scale. (These are potentially serious or fatal risks that the public recognizes could happen but, using their own life experiences as a guide, folks don't really go out of their way to avoid.)

The patient can then use this "home-base zone as a context for evaluating the likelihood of some new or unfamiliar risk. (**Figure 6.**)

> *Tell me and I'll forget;*
> *Show me and I may remember;*
> *Involve me and I will understand.*
>
> — *Modified from Confucius*

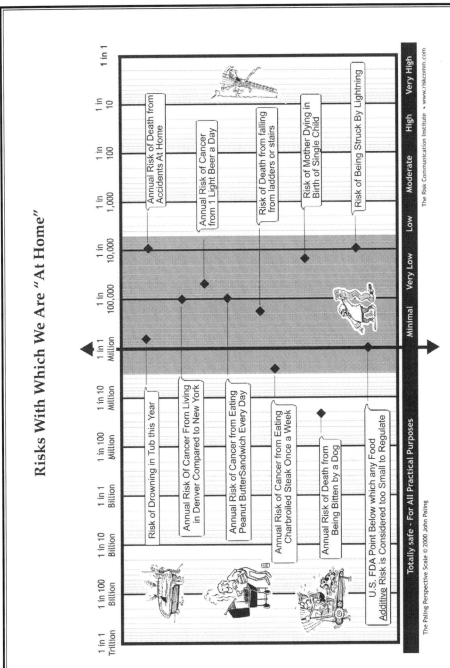

Figure 6: A perspective scale showing the zone of risks that most people are "at home with"

Throughout the developed world, the public's "comfort zone" occurs at likelihood levels of 1 in 10,000 down to 1 in 10 million and less. This is *not* dependent on one single comparative frame of reference.

7. Use visual aids as tools to reinforce relationships with patients.

Sharing visual aids provides opportunities to demonstrate competence and caring and thus optimize the patient's acceptance of the doctor's information.

It would be difficult to find a tool more beneficial for communicating numbers associated with health risks than a visual aid. They are effective, time saving tools that increase the patient's chance of understanding risks. However they also offer another benefit that is almost as important. They serve as a wonderfully effective (and inexpensive) bridge that leads to deepening the bond of partnership between patients and doctors. At the same time, they positively support the healing relationship by:

- encouraging the likelihood of a positive outcome,

- allowing space for the placebo effect to work, and also

- optimizing the likelihood that the doctor's factual information about risks will be "heard" and influence the patients' decisions.

Each one of these outcomes on its own is a hugely important benefit. Together they take the old methods of risk communication to new levels. The sense of caring and "being on the side of the patient" is enhanced if the doctor takes a palette or a perspective scale and sits down and shares information that is of crucial concern to that particular person.

> *In the last analysis, what we ARE communicates far more eloquently than anything we SAY*
>
> — *www.brightquotes.com*

USING VISUAL AIDS CAN MAKE DOCTORS FEEL LIKE HEROES

Doctors are widely respected and admired by society, however, they sometimes feel dissatisfaction knowing that they aren't getting through to their patients as well as they would like. Now, in the area of risk communication at least, they can feel the professional satisfaction of knowing that their patients are being given the best possible chance of understanding the numbers while keeping their focus on the positive possibilities for their future.

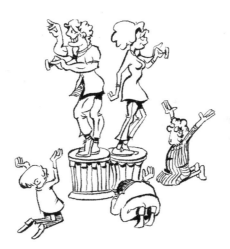

Turning mere mortals into superstars.

SECTION TWO

THE CHALLENGES

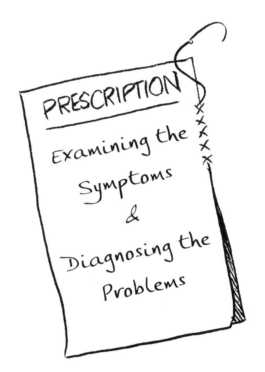

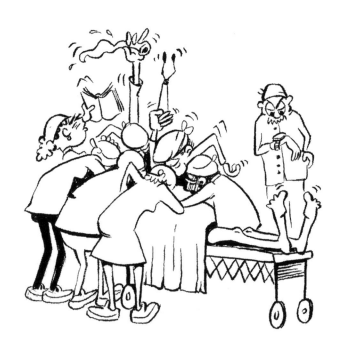

*At med school, there's no time for teaching
topics like risk communication.*

2

13 REASONS WHY GOOD DOCTORS STRUGGLE TO ACHIEVE PATIENT UNDERSTANDING

"Patients just don't get it..."

Helping patients understand risks is a routine responsibility for millions of healthcare professionals in all types of specialties. For a start, it is the essence of all informed consent and all genetic counseling. It is also pivotal to discussing medication side effects and the consequences of unhealthy lifestyles – as well as a response to the endless health scares reported by the media. Yet despite the fact that risk communication is such a familiar part of the job, it is rarely as successful as it might be – not only for the patient but also for the personal and professional interests of the doctor. The process is never uniform. There is no single "best practice" to deal with all patients alike; and knowing the facts is only one part of the equation.

In reality, the process is complicated by all the emotional, practical and legal judgments that may be involved. Thus, before we move on to introduce the toolbox of strategies to help patients understand risks, it is useful to start out by listing some of the reasons why good doctors often struggle as they try to explain risks to patients. Only then can the reasons behind many of our later recommendations be fully understood.

It is convenient to divide the many factors that can obstruct successful doctor-patient communication into four broad categories:

CHALLENGES INHERENT IN THE HEALTHCARE SYSTEM

1. Modern healthcare can be very complex with many overlapping issues that are hard to simplify for patients.

Physicians understand the complexities and time pressures of modern medicine and, accordingly, realize that full explanations are rarely practical or expected. Inevitably, risk communication becomes much simplified and usually results in only a limited amount of information about the most immediate and troubling side effects being offered.

2. Doctors do not get the chance to learn from experts in risk communication from other professions.

All doctors undergo very lengthy training but, with so much biomedical information to absorb, there is no time for teaching topics like effective risk communication. However, other professions have studied this field extensively yet many of their lessons have never found their way into clinical practice.

Interestingly, we find that most doctors develop an interest in the topic after they have established a reputation in their chosen field.

3. The legally approved requirements for communicating risks support the status quo – not change.

The law varies somewhat from place to place but typically it requires only that doctors "communicate risks in a manner that is consistent with what is currently carried out within the profession." (In Florida, "no recovery shall be allowed . . . when consent . . . was in accordance with an accepted standard of medical practice among members of the medical profession with similar training . . .")

This means that if a doctor's performance meets the current norm for the profession, then he is unlikely to be found guilty of inadequate informed consent. This limits incentives to improve and is just one of several ways in which possible malpractice exposure influences the way risk communication is carried out.

4. Sometimes, informed consent is focused more on protecting doctors and hospitals from legal challenges rather than on providing understanding for patients.

It is hard to blame the profession for this. In the U.S. particularly, this is a practical way of managing risks from the ever-present threat of malpractice claims. I think it is fair to point out that, although there is no doubt that the primary purpose of establishing informed consent requirements was to protect the patient, it is notable that in practice it is the patient who signs the form, not the doctor!

PROBLEMS ARISING FROM LIMITATIONS AND ATTITUDES OF PATIENTS

5. Patients often don't have the necessary education to understand the facts about risks.

This is a challenge for doctor-patient communication throughout the world. I will quote some American figures here but it is important to recognize that, for the purpose of this list, the numbers are not that different for many of the western countries.

Approximately 47% of the adult public has been defined as either illiterate or marginally literate in English and over 20% test at or below the lowest level of literacy and numeracy.[1,2] Then, to get a feel for the magnitude of this daily challenge for doctors, add in the inevitable difficulties of communication with patients who are not fluent in English (or whatever other languages the doctor uses), or who are mentally impaired or who simply have difficulties in comprehension because of advanced age.

Given these numbers, it is not surprising that many patients will have great difficulty understanding the data presented to them and will easily be confused by percentages and probabilities.

6. Patients let their emotions dominate their assessment of risks.

This is regularly listed as the number one challenge when we ask doctors, "What is the biggest obstacle you have in getting your patients to understand risks?" In view of its importance, this topic is given special attention in this book.

Now we have established that there are a lot of patients who simply lack the formal education to understand much detail about their risks, it might be expected that these are the people will inevitably make their medical decisions based on their emotions. However, perhaps surprisingly, this is only part of the story. It is now clear that patients at all educational levels always involve their own emotions in evaluating risks. Thus, doctors may find all kinds of patients can be influenced as much by unqualified neighbors and friends as by the logic of the medical facts about risks.

7. Patients differ very widely in their wishes for involvement.

Despite the ethical ideal of patient autonomy, many patients still prefer that their doctor recommends the medical decisions best for them. At the other extreme, there are many patients – and particularly family members responsible for a loved one – who have a voracious appetite to learn all they can before they make a decision. And because of the diversity of human nature, there is every gradation in between.

As might be expected, the more serious the illness, the more likely it is that patients want their doctor to make the decision for them. Also, older patients have less desire than younger patients to make their own medical decisions.[3]

Because many patients just want the doctor to decide for them, it would be easy to assume that patients don't really want information about their risks. However, research shows that there is no correlation between the desire for information and the desire for decision-making. In fact, a vast majority of patients declare a strong interest in being well informed even if they then readily hand over decision-making to their doctor. This has been described as "paternalism with permission." [3]

8. Patients may hold unrealistic expectations of "miracle medicine."

Doctors today are just one source of information for patients and they may no longer be the most influential.

Some patients are so eager to believe in the blessings of modern medicine that they may not be willing to "hear" the risks that their doctor tells them about. Patients can be over-optimistic, not accept the uncertainties and, in turn, may be more likely to react in disappointment and anger if the benefits they are expecting don't materialize. Consumers with unrealistic expectations are often harder to please and, as we might expect, more ready to sue.

When the media reports on medical advances in glowing terms, it can easily lead some patients to believe that there is now a "miracle medicine" or a proven procedure for every problem. This tendency is reinforced by numerous offers of alternative treatments available on the internet. To the desperate or indiscriminating patients, this can give the impression that if you just look long enough, some angel is going to pop out and seductively offer medical miracles.

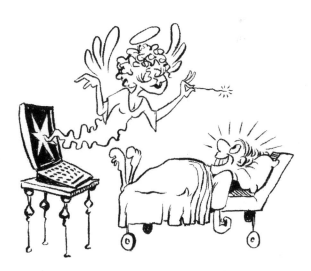

Miracle cures from the web.

9. The massive increase of data available to patients can lead to doctors' judgments being questioned.

Some patients feel that their busy doctor might not be familiar with all the newest information so, fortified by their recent readings from the internet, they openly (or insidiously) challenge their physician's judgment. Such an assertive attitude is fueled by the American pharmaceutical industry's marketing trend: "Ask your doctor about whether our product is right for you."

Without a doubt, effective risk communication is much harder – or near impossible – to achieve if the patient doesn't trust her doctor to have all the facts about her condition.

CHALLENGES THAT ONLY DOCTORS EXPERIENCE

10. There can be great uncertainty when estimating the levels of the risk for a particular patient.

One of the greatest difficulties in communicating risks is to overcome the patient's wish to be told certainties about their individual situation. Doctors of course know that outcomes can vary greatly depending on preexisting conditions and various other complicating factors and, because of this, physicians can sometimes only give best guesses.

This doesn't stop patients wanting to hear risks categorized in a safe / unsafe dichotomy. It is almost as if they crave that unambiguous clarity in order to simplify their task of making their risk decisions.

Some procedures now come with a well documented history that permits the doctor to quote firm likelihoods of a successful outcome. Others, such as clinical trials and some major surgeries, don't.

Then again, there is the issue of how, if at all, doctors should explain test results to patients. Issues such as false positives or false negatives, and differing sensitivities of different tests all influence the predicted risk numbers. Doctors can sometimes calculate the patient's actual odds that take account of these imperfections of testing,[4] however, for practical purposes, this exercise is not called for.

The bottom line is that the spectrum of healthcare has a lot of uncertainties to communicate. At the end of the day, doctors do what they've always done. They do the best they can.

11. Uncertainty about how much detail to provide to patients.

At present, there is an uncomfortable disconnect between what unfettered ethical principles may suggest and what is realistic in practice. This can lead to skeptical thoughts such as, "How far do they expect me to go in listing the possible risks? For the surgery that I do, you'd need an encyclopedia."

Having studied the magnitudes and likelihoods of many types of different risks in society, I side with pragmatic doctors who try to make informed consent a meaningful but manageable process for their patients by dealing only with the most likely serious risks.

12. Not telling the full truth about risks may be in the patient's best interests.

In an effort to maintain an upbeat psychological state in their patients, doctors may consciously withhold discussion of possible risks and shade explanations of the potential outcomes. Some would strongly criticize this approach as "benign paternalism." Indeed, this approach may be counter productive given the new possibilities that now exist for positive risk communication. Others would argue that this deliberate strategy still represents a valuable tool in the art of medicine.

I have had one doctor ask me, "How can it help if I overload the patient with too many side effects?" Another pointed me to a quote from Oliver Wendell Holmes: "Your patient has no more right to all the truth you know than he has to all the medicine in your saddlebag."

Candidly, I don't have the answer. But I do know that well-meaning physicians frequently explain risks in ways that can needlessly frighten patients and this must work against the patients' interests. For these and many other reasons, I started this book with the heart-felt opinion that "Doctors have the most challenging job in all risk communication."

CHALLENGES THAT DOCTORS MAY NOT BE AWARE OF

13. The ways that most doctors explain risks can easily obstruct patient understanding.

This suggestion sometimes provokes a response like, "Don't insult me. I have been doing informed consents for years and do it perfectly well."

Maybe. However, this mind-set might be an impediment to effective communication if "doing it well" is only judged by the *feelings* of the doctor and not the *understanding* of the patient.

In the pages that follow, I will point out several ways in which current practices in the profession are likely to work against the best interests of patients. Once we have identified the patient's problems, we can move on to suggest our strategies and solutions.

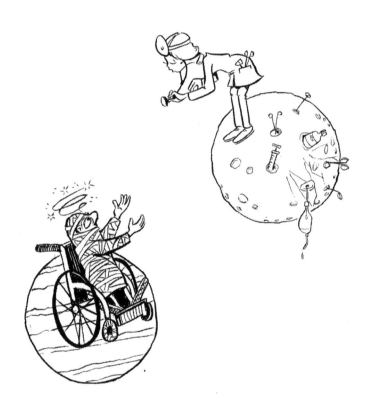

Might as well be living on different planets.

3

HOW DOCTORS AND PATIENTS SEE RISKS (AND MANY OTHER THINGS) DIFFERENTLY

Medics are from Mars and Patients are from Pluto!

Recently, a group of young doctors in England undertook a small research project as part of their training. Since it had been drummed into them that "the doctor-patient relationship is the most crucial aspect of effective patient care," they decided to investigate that topic in more detail. Among other things, they asked doctors and patients the simple question, "What, in your view, defines a good doctor?"

The results were revealing. The two parties answered a multiple choice questionnaire in consistently different ways. Specifically, the doctors stated that "diagnostic ability" was the most important quality of a good doctor, whereas patients said that "listening" was the most important thing. More strikingly, the skill that patients rated as the most important quality was placed last in line by the doctors themselves. Thus, instead of sharing basic values as might be expected in any successful partnership, the two parties' basic priorities seemed planets apart.

Although the study could not be claimed to be rigorous, its conclusion is supported by extensive studies published by the Association of American Medical Colleges in 1998[1] that also confirmed that the two parties rate things differently when judging the quality of a doctor. Good communication and caring are always paramount in the mind of the patient. For example, the top three categories for what most influences a patient's choice of a good doctor were "how well a doctor communicates with patients and shows a caring attitude" (85%); "explaining medical or technical procedures in a way that is easy to understand" (77%); "listening to you and taking the time to ask you more questions" (76%).

On the other hand, issues rated highly by doctors like "how many years in practice" and "whether doctor attended a well-known medical school" were far less important in the minds of patients (32% and 27% respectively).

A similar situation exists for pharmacists. Patients orientate more to the professional being "helpful" rather than "knowledgeable."[2]

EMOTIONAL FACTORS DOMINATE WHEN PATIENTS DECIDE WHAT MAKES A "GOOD DOCTOR"

When you stop to think about it, this should not be surprising. It is a natural outcome from the dichotomy of knowledge and experience of the two parties. Patients typically do not have the medical expertise to be able to judge the technical competence of their doctors so they are strongly impacted by their feelings about their doctor's level of care. In a way, this becomes a surrogate for trust and also for assessments of proficiency.

Healthcare professionals on the other hand, have many factual criteria for knowing how (technically) "good" any professional colleague is. Their evaluation of quality of performance and outcomes is likely to be the more accurate, so part of our challenge in this book is to optimize the opportunity for patients to really understand their doctor's information.

It is clear that health professionals and patients do see certain things differently. This does not just apply to their differing definitions of a good doctor but also when it comes to rating healthcare risks.

EMOTIONAL FACTORS ALSO DOMINATE WHEN PATIENTS DECIDE WHAT IS A "BIG RISK"

Here again, professionals focus on the facts. After all, evidence-based medicine is the mark of the professional. Patients, on the other hand, make their judgments based on their own emotional filters. This can cause doctors to despair when the medical facts clearly show something is in their patient's best interests yet this doesn't translate to appropriate actions and decisions. The doctor's natural response then is to seek better ways of laying out the data or providing more statistics. This might work if, in fact, their patients primarily made their medical choices by reviewing the evidence. However, they don't.

There is now an extensive body of social science knowledge that shows that the public does not think rationally about risks.[3] There is a tendency for people to overestimate the dangers and undervalue the benefits. So, when it comes to communicating risks, doctors cannot avoid the reality that patients are going to process the data in their brains and that their decisions can have as much to do with feelings as the numbers. This presents such profound challenges for doctors that it is worth spending a few moments on the implications.

First, this is not a situation that is caused by limitations of education. In fact, recent publications[4] suggest that this filtering is true not just for patients but for all people, including doctors, particularly when they have to make decisions in areas where they are not experts. Hence, when doctors decide whom to marry, what job to take, how much money to risk, they too allow their forebrain to filter the facts through value judgments. This puts them in a comparable situation to most patients considering their risks. Current thinking is that there are not two separate worlds – emotions and logical thought. The facts are *always* filtered through the emotions so the challenge for doctors is to optimize the chance that the data that they present to patients will get an objective "hearing."

Secondly, this primacy of the emotional over the factual makes total sense in an evolutionary context, too. In ancestral times, humans were surrounded on every side by risks – many of them imminent, sudden and serious. In such circumstances, the likelihood of personal harm from a possible threat would best be measured by previous personal experiences and the emotional responses of neighbors. This basic domination of feelings over facts has the added advantage that it is far quicker to make decisions this way – another reason why it suited our ancestors so well and hence why we are now predisposed to operate the same way too.

When you think about it, if our tribal ancestors were to survive, they all needed to be hard wired to quickly assess risks in those centuries before there were any factual records to serve as a basis for making estimates. In that light, it is not surprising that various "panic factors" were evolved. They make ideal guidelines for protecting an individual in the pre-technology age.

In our modern technologically advanced age, the same "emotional filter process" makes just as much sense. There is simply no time to logically weigh all the options of the huge volume of decisions that each of us makes every day. Over our lifetime, each of us has become our own personal risk assessor and, for the most part, our judgments are likely to be made without an analytical consideration of the facts.

The message for doctors from this is clear. Risk communication is far more effective when the patient's emotions are seen as legitimate.

It is natural that this can be somewhat frustrating for doctors who, after all, have been trained to put aside their feelings, interpret data logically and make evidence-based decisions. Yet, when they confront the reality of how the human body actually functions (as all doctors must), physicians come to recognize that successful risk communication is far more than finding ways to simplify medical information. In fact, patients will resist even a superb factual communication showing only low risks when they don't totally trust their doctor or feel frightened, or angry or powerless.

FACTORS LIKELY TO CAUSE THE PUBLIC'S PERCEPTION OF A RISK TO BE EXAGGERATED

We can explain some of the apparently "illogical" responses that patients may appear to display when we recognize the power and influence of the public's emotional filters.

Researchers working on risk communication in other fields have been able to identify about a dozen different factors that, if present, cause a particular risk to be perceived as large or small *almost independently of the facts of likelihood and consequences.*[5, 6.]

It turns out that *some types of risks* are likely to have an increased emotional impact. And *whether the risk communicator is trusted* can impact the perceived seriousness of the risk.

What sort of risk it is

Here is a list of some of the *types* of risks that are likely to make the general public exaggerate the perception of fear. (The term in brackets shows what is less likely to cause an excessive response.)

Involuntary (as opposed to voluntary)
Think of fears of industrial pollution exposure vs. dangerous sports or smoking.

Industrial (as opposed to natural)
Think of minute levels of pesticide residues vs. organic foods and "pure" bottled waters.

Unfamiliar (as opposed to familiar)
Think of genetically modified foods vs. junk foods.

Catastrophic (as opposed to chronic)
Think if a year's worth of deaths attributed to smoking occurred on just one day instead of being chronically spread through the year.

Particularly dreaded (as opposed to not dreaded)

Think of the reaction to "cancer" vs. pneumonia

Unfair (as opposed to fair)

Think of death as a result of drunk driver vs. death from a falling tree.

Lack of control (as opposed to keeping control)

Think of feeling pressured to take a particular treatment vs. the ability to decide for yourself among various options.

Once doctors become aware of the potential for these types of risks to diminish (or exaggerate) the public's perception of risk, it is easy to apply them to healthcare issues.[3] Thus, risks from smoking, overeating, excessive alcohol and unprotected sex are often perceived by patients to be "not that big" because they don't trigger the emotional fear factors. More particularly, these risks are chronic and not dreaded. The behavior that causes them is familiar and voluntary – and the patient is in control (at least they are not coerced by others).

Using the same filter, we could predict in advance that genetically modified foods would generate great fear just because they are "industrial" (rather than natural), the technology is totally unfamiliar (as opposed to familiar) and the public felt that they or other living things might get "involuntarily" exposed.

Who tells you

Here are three (oversimplified) images of the doctor that can cause patients to exaggerate the perception of risk. (The first category in each case is what is likely to provoke excessive fear.)

Limited trust in the communicator

(as opposed to total trust)

Marginally responsive communicator

(as opposed to totally responsive)

Doubts about total commitment

(as opposed to totally on the side of the patient)

Trust stands out as one of the most powerful and influential of all those factors that affect a person's rating of their risks – whatever type of concerns they have. Clearly, this is something that already exists in large measure in most doctor-patient relationships. After all, patients clearly "entrust" doctors with their health – often literally putting their lives in their hands. Doctors can rightly claim that patients certainly do respect and trust the competence of a noble profession and, indeed, are enormously grateful for the professional services they receive.

Nonetheless, when it comes to effective risk communication, the sense of trust that influences a patient's perception of risks is more personal. It reflects more than individual or institutional competence. The patient's sense of trust involves a significant element of *the feeling* of caring alongside *the fact* of competence.

My associate John Spence, a nationally known leadership consultant, summarizes this point elegantly in a powerful visual. It shows the permutations of different levels of competence and caring.

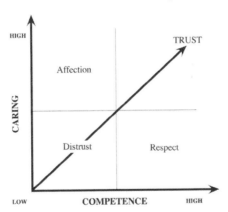

Figure 2: The Quadrants of Trust
(after John Spence with permission)

- Low competence and low caring are the hallmarks of Distrust.
- High caring could be lavishly delivered with low competence—and as a result be potentially fatal. Such a combination would generate the reaction of Affection.
- High competence alone with little or no sense of caring gives, not Trust but Respect.
- It is only when there is a high blend of Competence and Caring that the patient feels real Trust on a personal level.

The *Wall Street Journal*,[7] in an article reporting on how doctors themselves find a good doctor ended with a quote from a urologist: "Personally speaking, the most important thing is trust in a physician and being able to communicate with him or her in good times and bad."

In reality, we all know that it is totally false to talk of doctors as being *either* caring *or* competent. The vast majority of course are both. But the point I want to make is that typically patients take a doctor's *professionalism* for granted whereas doctors take their *caring* for granted. My suggestion is that this dichotomy can be the basis of misunderstandings and that, as the professionals in the partnership, it is up to doctors to be aware of the challenge and to take the initiative to overcome it.

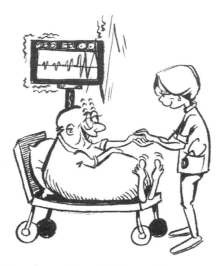

Patients always have their sensitive antennae
tuned for caring.

In this book, we will offer some simple tools that not only *help doctors with the communication of data about risks but, just as important, serve to facilitate the bonding process* between doctors and patients, in this way optimizing the patient's sense of trust. We recommend thinking of visual aids as valuable "social lubricants" -- the term used by behaviorists to describe the way pet owners bond easily with other humans when they are with their companion animals.

Sharing visual aids can provide a similar lubrication of the relationship – just as when individuals share anything in a social setting.

THE MAGIC MOMENT

As a patient, I feel uniquely vulnerable and crave a lot of reassurance when I learn that I have been diagnosed as having something wrong with me and then am told what my risks and choices are. At that moment, doctors have a golden opportunity to demonstrate both competence and caring by the way they deal with the informational and emotional needs of patients. In my opinion, there is no better time for establishing trust. It is then that doctors should not only convey their knowledge and invite discussion but also consciously make deposits into what Stephen Covey[8] calls the "emotional bank account" of caring.

And yet, tragically, these explanations of risks are often debased into largely perfunctory formalities and dispiriting legal requirements. As a result, informed consent largely passes as a neglected opportunity – a missed magic moment.

From my perspective at the periphery of much of the healthcare system, it grieves me to find such a massive disconnect between those who approach informed consent from a purely theoretical basis and those who have the practical responsibility for making it work. Equally, I am saddened by the fact that, when it comes to risk communication, some healthcare organizations focus primarily on minimizing exposure to medical malpractice claims – rather than most effectively informing patients.

This emphasis is perhaps not at all surprising, given the trauma and costs of med malpractice claims and the institutional responsibilities of hospital risk managers and defense attorneys. However, this book makes the case that when doctors bond with patients by such practices as working together and sharing simple visual communication tools, the exposure to malpractice claims should also be reduced. (See p. 154.)

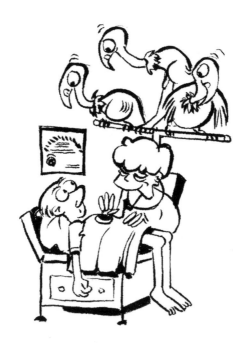

*Like it or not, lawyers' attention to the profession
can be a powerful stimulant for change.*

4

THE FORCES FOR CHANGE

A Bird in the Hand Can Mess Up Your Wrist.

Ifyou hold on to something for too long, it may backfire on you!

In this chapter, I will argue that this applies not just to the avian world but also to the way that most healthcare organizations inform patients about their risks. In my opinion, what currently gets by as adequate informed consent is due for a change. Here's why:

The old approach of "just do whatever is typical in the profession" will not hold up in the face of cumulative research that clearly shows the inadequacies of the present system. Also, I happen to believe that once doctors become aware that they can increase the level of understanding for, at the very minimum, 25% of their patients with negligible extra time or money, then they will embrace the opportunities in the spirit of their calling. In addition, there are some needlessly troublesome weak links in the status quo.

- Risk communication as it is commonly practiced often doesn't work.
- Patients are not being provided with "information" prior to giving their supposedly "informed" consent.

- Doctors often don't tell patients about all the risks that are more than "minimal." (I don't blame them. This expectation also needs reexamining)
- Proven best practices from other professions have been reported in the major journals but have not been adopted into healthcare.
- Institutions and drug companies like to claim that they are patient-focused yet in practice have not adopted solutions to overcome the known obstacles to patient understanding.
- Adversarial lawyers could reasonably claim that accepting the status quo implies a lack of care for the best interests of patients.

These allegations obviously merit some justification so let me go through them one by one. Notice first that I do not claim that such deficiencies are universal but rather that they not uncommon, that they are needless and that with effectively no extra time and money, the patients' interests could be better served. In aggregate, I suggest the factors are in place to drive change.

1. Many patients have wildly inaccurate perceptions of their levels of risk after their doctor has explained the facts to them.

This has been clearly demonstrated in a variety of disciplines but none more so than in heart patients. A recent high-profile inquiry by the U.K. General Medical Council found that patients were clearly misinformed about the risk associated with heart surgery.[1]

Another British study concluded that carotid endarterectomy patients simply "failed to understand the risks and benefits associated with CEA" having been told them by their surgeon.[2]

In a careful cross-sectional study of myocardial infarction patients in New Zealand, it was found that patients' risk perceptions showed no relationship to the Thrombosis in Myocardial Infarction (TMI) risk scores that the patients had been told about.[3]

In layman's terms, these erroneous perceptions could not be related to age, gender, family history of heart disease, previous MI, diabetics or smoking. In other words, "in-patient hospital care appears to be unsuccessful in effectively communicating prognosis to patients."

Since patients' perception of the risks of a future attack can be a powerful motivating factor in making their medical decisions, this failure of communication is far more than an academic issue.

2. Currently most informed consents typically do NOT provide "information." Instead, they provide "data," which is a very different thing.

Most doctors readily agree that data and information are not the same. Even in common usage they carry different levels of meaning. This is no surprise to professional communicators who have been taught to recognize them as progressive levels of communication. "Data" are raw facts or statistics. "Information" on the other hand is *"data presented in a context* that makes it meaningful to the recipient."

This distinction is very relevant to risk communication for it means that *providing information* is not just about presenting facts and numbers but *also requires that a meaningful context is presented too.*

Taking a simple example, if you tell a 60-year-old man he has a PSA reading of 10, you are imparting only data. It is not until you add that "any figure over 3 is considered to be of concern" that you move toward allowing the patient to put the data into a meaningful context thus moving the communication into providing "information."

When it comes to explaining the likelihood of different treatment options, doctors most commonly express the risk numbers in terms of the odds. For example: "There's about a 1 in 400 chance that it may result in death." Again, such odds remain "data" until some context is provided. Alternate options and their estimated outcomes would help, as would a way of showing patients what level of likelihood 1 in 400 represents in other areas of their life's experiences. (Perhaps that the annual risk of dying from accidental poisoning is 1 in 400.[4])

Again, only when you deliver context do you truly deliver information—which is, after all, the whole intention of the concept of informed consent. Much risk communication does not give meaningful context or perspective, hence it does not provide information.

3. Most informed consents do not introduce patients to all the risks that are "more than minimal" as is required by U.S. Food & Drug Administration Guidelines

Until recently, "minimal risk" used to be a conveniently vague concept. However, in 2001 America's National Bioethics Advisory Commission[5] recommended how minimal risks should be defined.

In essence, they defined "minimal" in terms of routine events such as "driving to work, crossing the street, getting a blood test or answering questions over the phone." This means we can now put numbers to these events and the practical consequences of defining "minimal" in this way could mean that any risk more likely than 1 in 10 million should be declared to patients.

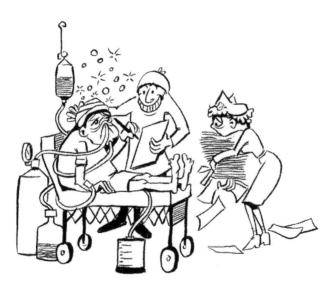

Patients should be told "all risks greater than minimal".

Most healthcare providers would see such a standard as being blatantly impracticable. For many operations, this would mean listing hundreds of infinitely remote possibilities. Obviously, the threshold required for informed consent should be redefined along far more realistic grounds.

If nothing else, someone might question why the level of medical errors estimated by the Institute of Medicine[6] does not feature in informed consents. The likelihood for those iatrogenic risks is many orders of magnitude greater than those risks mentioned by the bioethics advisory commission – yet are seemingly not mentioned.

Those of us in risk communication have recognized for a long time that there is often a disconnect between theoretical considerations and what really goes on in clinical practice. This can lead to one undesirable consequence. *If standards are set at a level that the folk who have to carry them out know are impracticable, it actually discourages people from trying to improve on the status quo.* Unattainable goals provide no motivation to improve.

Putting all this together, I will simply add "Impractical definitions of minimal risks" as another reason why risk communication in healthcare is due for a change

4. Best practices from other professions have not been adopted into healthcare.

The *British Medical Journal* has led the major journals by publishing a special edition devoted to communicating risks.[7] In addition, there are many articles in specialist medical publications for those with an interest in learning more about the topic as well as books about risk communication in non-healthcare arenas. However, because this is a field few are actively concerned about, the suggested solutions to overcome patients' problems have not been widely adopted in clinical practice. However, reviews of at least some existing patient education materials conclude that "a new generation of materials is needed."[8]

I hope this book will help increase the level of awareness of the deficiencies of the status quo as well as the available solutions.

5. Institutions claiming to be patient-focused will be particularly vulnerable to challenges.

Once patient-focused institutions become aware of the counter-productive effects of many of the common ways of communicating risks, then some changes from the status quo become inevitable. Just as it would be unacceptable for healthcare professionals to not use readily available tools to improve patient care in surgery, so too should it be unacceptable to not use the most effective communications tools for something as fundamental as discussing risks with patients.

I believe that we can start a movement towards improvement just by increasing awareness of how simple visual aids can significantly help patients.

Realistically, the most powerful stimulus for change will come when there is a body of independent research that reinforces the value of new approaches to patient communication. This would lead to the acceptance of new "best practices" within the profession and then strategies such as those in this book will become mainstream.

We are a long way from this at present but this book is intended to serve as a catalyst for clinicians in all disciplines to try out some of the strategies for themselves.

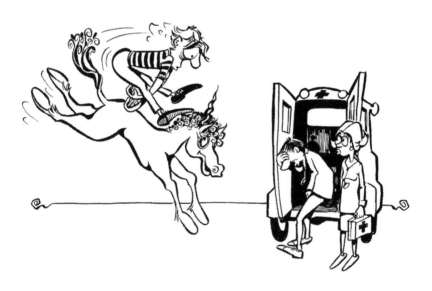

Never Play Leapfrog with a Unicorn!

5

BAD POINTS ABOUT CURRENT PRACTICES

Never play leapfrog with a unicorn

It is tempting for experienced doctors to believe that the old, traditional ways of communicating risks to patients work just fine. As such, it may be irritating to be confronted with evidence that, in practice, the most common ways that doctors explain risks can now be seen as flawed and capable of easy improvement. This chapter sets out to provide evidence for this claim as a prelude to considering alternatives.

WHY A "SMALL OPERATION" IS ALWAYS DONE ON SOMEONE ELSE!

There is always the possibility of misunderstandings when people from two cultures set out to work together. Although not much has been written about it, there is convincing research that shows that although doctors and patients may use identical words, the meaning that comes across the cultural divide can be totally different from what was intended.

There is a lot of evidence for this including one influential paper analyzing the legal records that were parts of med malpractice cases in the U.S. The research looked at over 450 cases in all 50 states over a 40-year period. It demonstrated a persistent disconnect between the intended levels of likelihood communicated by the clinicians and what was actually understood by the patients.[1]

Naturally, a doctor knows perfectly well what he means when he categorizes a risk in descriptive terms. However, if he is unaware that descriptive terms convey *only the perspective of the person using them,* he will be misleading himself if he believes that his patient has been properly "informed." It is pretty obvious that, if the patient doesn't have the healthcare professional's knowledge and context, all such descriptive words are likely to mean widely different things to different patients.

These levels of disparity are not trivial, particularly when you consider the most common descriptors, such as "a low risk." We investigated this on our web site. We outlined a simple medical consultation scenario and invited readers to indicate the level of likelihood that was intended by "a low risk." We found that some individuals interpreted it as meaning odds as high as 1 in 5, while others said they would expect the term to be used for odds of 1 in 10,000. It all depends on people's knowledge – or expectations – of the context.

Remember: No context = No information

PURELY DESCRIPTIVE TERMS DON'T WORK

The key finding from these examples is that purely descriptive terms simply don't work when it comes to accurately communicating likelihoods to patients.

Despite this, the vast majority of doctors throughout the world (and Institutional Review Boards in the U.S.) continue to define the level of risks for their patients purely with these descriptive terms.

Patients can hear a wide vocabulary of familiar terms int explain their risks. Words such as negligible, high, moderate, minimal, likely, severe, remote, mild are multiplied by such qualifiers as very, rather, extremely, quite or sometimes... and so on. Similarly side effects for drugs or treatments may be rare, common, possible, frequent, or uncommon.

Because patients use these familiar words themselves and know what *they* mean by them, they are likely to assume that the doctor means the same thing. Unfortunately this may not be the case, and unintentionally many patients may leave an encounter with their doctor to some degree "misinformed."[2]

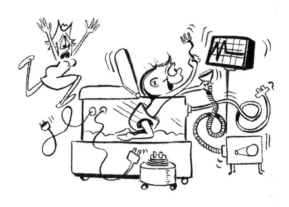

A Low Risk?

RELATIVE RISKS

Another common source of miscommunication is when doctors, drug companies, government agencies and the media inform members of the public about a particular issue in terms of relative risks. Doctors are totally comfortable hearing research results expressed in this way. Patients, on the other hand, live in a different world and can totally misunderstand what the numbers appear to be saying.

If you accept that "information" is data given along with a context that the patient can relate to – then it is immediately obvious that statements of relative risk do not qualify. The numbers are effectively meaningless unless the listener happens to be an expert and know the baseline level of risk that is being used for comparison.

To make matters even worse, medical agencies and regulators have not taken a stand to demand consistency in how the profession explains risk numbers to patients. This can result in almost comically differing statements about the size of the identical risk.

For example, let's say that the records show that about 2 out of 100 people of a defined population are at risk of having a heart attack over the next 5 years. However, other studies may have shown that if the patient takes a daily aspirin over that time, the risk will be lowered so that the odds would be that only 1 person out of 100 hundred would be likely to have a heart attack.

You could hardly imagine a simpler risk communication scenario. Yet one doctor might tell the patient, "Aspirin reduces your risk of heart attack by 1% while another doctor (using the same data) might say "Aspirin reduces your risk by 50%." Yet despite this obvious source of confusion, different doctors could claim that their way of expressing the results was right.

The first doctor would be accurate in that he meant "the risk would normally be 2% but aspirin reduces those odds down to 1%." (A 1% reduction – a statement of *absolute* risk.)

But the second doctor would also be accurate, as he simply meant to communicate that, if you take aspirin, the risk is now halved; down from 2% to 1%. (This is a statement of *relative* risk.)

From the point of view of patient understanding, however, this potential for confusion cries out for a solution. When doctors, agencies and reporters communicate with patients and the public, expressions of relative risks should be outlawed. A truly patient-focused profession should define and reinforce a clear policy to help patients understand the absolute numbers that relate to their conditions.

Then, to further reinforce the importance of this opinion, there is the additional issue of how using relative risks gives patients surprisingly exaggerated impressions of what the actual numbers show. Health professionals are usually well aware of this.

For example, if patients were told in terms of relative risks that some new drug "showed a 50% improvement over a previous one," most of them would believe that it represented a vast improvement. However, in a situation with 1000 patients, a 50% improvement could mean nothing more than, instead of only two patients being cured, three were. Hypothetically that could still mean that 997 were likely to die – hardly a major breakthrough, even with the improved treatment.

Sadly, the media, drug companies and healthcare agencies still present risks in relative terms and, from this, the numbers get into the minds of doctors and patients. For example, in 2002 the press reported[3] research findings that claimed that hormone replacement therapy had been found to cause "a 26% increase risk of breast cancer, a 41% increased risk of stroke and a 29% risk of heart attack and cardiac death."

Since these reports of changes in health effects related to harmful scenarios, patients naturally quit taking such treatments. Even those women who still desperately wanted the intended benefits would naturally avoid choices where the risks seemed so high.

If the risks had been expressed in a more objective way using absolute numbers, the level of panic would have been much lower. For example, the actual increased risk of breast cancer as a result of taking HT for a 5-year period is estimated at 4 women per thousand. In other words, 996 out of the thousand could be expected to receive the benefits and not suffer an increased cancer risk. Such a factual statement of the actual numbers is likely to produce a different reaction on the part of the typical patient.

If new research shows relatively small changes in the absolute numbers in a negative direction, patients become deeply disillusioned. What they had thought were massively helpful and safe products are suddenly cast as unexpected threats to their health. A crisis of trust and confusion washes over patients and corporate profits get swept away. When this happens, you might think that drug companies would want to have the results expressed as absolute numbers so that patients would not take away an exaggerated impression. But it is not as simple as that.

In the same way that statements of relative risks can make a drug appear a poor choice when the numbers are negative, the same approach can result in small absolute improvements appearing as massive breakthroughs when expressed in this format. Understandably, this is hard for marketing departments for commercial products to resist.

Doctors should keep in mind that when patients arrive with a self-diagnosed opinion about their problem or their treatment, they may well have exaggerated expectations that come from having heard the risks or benefits expressed in relative terms from the media. *If the doctor does not correct this impression, it is very likely that the patient will make her healthcare choices according to a skewed understanding of the true facts.* As we will see later, absolute numbers expressed on visual aids provide the best of all worlds.

Again it all comes down to information being data provided in a context that is meaningful to the patient. On this basis, I believe that relative risks should be banned from communications with patients.

I also strongly support those who have suggested that medical journals and readers should demand that risk always be expressed in absolute numbers as a condition of publication.[4]

FRAMING

Here is one more example of how the way most doctors communicate risks can work against their patients' best interests. Unless they are alert to the trap, doctors can unwittingly be led into a mind-set whereby they excessively scare their patients and actually bias them against perfectly sound medical decisions. Again let me explain. . .

Patients typically confront their doctor with their minds focused on learning from the expert about their possible risks. In response, the conscientious doctor might say something like, "Your chances of (experiencing a bad outcome) are around 3% or three in a hundred."

Such absolute numbers are perfectly clear but this scenario ignores what we know about the way people intuitively respond to the possibility of risks. A patient is likely to turn down a procedure where *the possibility of harm or failure* is predicted at, say, 3 out of 100 dying whereas the same procedure will be found acceptable if the odds are expressed as 97 out of 100 surviving or being cured.

A similar situation shows up from studies on the main factors influencing patients to take up or accept a particular treatment. Here too, the focus tends to be on avoiding the loss. For example, patients will decide to accept a treatment more out of fear of the possible negative outcomes rather than the improved mental comfort and the other benefits that might be predicted if they do.[5] A specific example is that when women were told they had a 20% chance of having a child with Down's syndrome (framed negatively) they were more likely to have an amniocentesis than if the risk were framed positively—an 80% chance of no abnormality.

The human brain seems to be hard-wired such that it responds more strongly to the possible negative outcomes than the positive ones. This again is possibly an adaptation from ancestral times where the need to be alert to – and avoid – unnecessary hazards was a prime filter for making survival decisions. The tendency still persists in the disproportionate power of negative advertising in political campaigns and the profound effect that a culture of fear has in changing the responsiveness of populations.

Once doctors understand that their patients are likely to make different choices according to how the likelihood numbers are framed, they will see the reasoning behind one of our later recommendations.

SPIN AND EUPHEMISMS

I cannot write about communicating risks without honestly addressing these other possible ways of biasing the opinions and decisions of patients.

Whenever I address this topic, I immediately think back to frenetic discussions with a client who begged me to substitute the word "casualties" for "deaths" in my public pronouncements. After a flurry of exchanges, the reason for the request was flushed out in print: "Because the euphemism doesn't sound quite so final."

All communicators have the ability to alter the tone of the message by the choice of words they use. There is nothing new in this. It is already well established as part of the armory of professionals in advertising, public relations and, of course, politics.

The option to spin the message is also available to people who talk about risks. It brings with it one additional responsibility for doctors (as if they needed any more.) Do not think that this "shading" of risk communications does not occur throughout healthcare too – particularly where important financial or political decisions may be influenced.

Hochhauser[6] has suggested that "spin" is commonly involved when patients are recruited for clinical trials. He points out that consent forms usually avoid using the word "experiment or experimental"— instead referring to "study, research investigation, trial or clinical research program." He speculates that patients would be less willing to sign up if they thought of it as an experiment since, in the minds of volunteers, "there are more risks in an experiment than in a study." Similarly, despite offering patients access to the "latest and most promising treatments" rarely is it made clear that, according to the FDA, about four out of five of the drugs in clinical trials will never get to market and that most subjects will not benefit from most clinical trials.

I have heard of other situations where doctors might deliberately "shade" the facts in their own interests. I was introduced to this early in my career when a questioner from my audience told me that, at medical school, they had been taught to exaggerate the risks when talking to patients so that, if things went badly, then at least the patient and her family had been warned, and they could prepare themselves. On the other hand, if things went well, the medical staff would come out as heroes!

I have problems with this. For me, this crosses the line for the simple reason that, at its root, such a practice is done mainly in the interests of the doctor and not those of the patient.

DEALING WITH POTENTIAL CONFLICTS

My guiding principle throughout this book is to encourage truly patient-focused risk communication. I have tried to show clinicians how to present risk data in the most neutral way possible while keeping a focus on their patients' best interests. In my opinion, one of the major strategies for achieving this is to always ensure that patients are shown the positive framing of their odds as well as the negative possibilities. This way, the physician shares the truth while helping maintain a basis for real hope.

That said, I am well aware that healthcare professionals occasionally do spin the way they present their knowledge to patients. They may "soften the message" for humanitarian reasons, hoping to spare their patient's feelings or in the belief that it will encourage a positive attitude. Alternatively, they may "color" the factual data in the hope that the patient will make a decision that supports what the doctor believes is best for that patient.

Some would argue that this is the very essence of why patients entrust themselves to their doctors in the first place. Others would claim that this paternal approach is no longer acceptable or indeed necessary now we know more about how patients deal with risks.

It is issues such as this that make risk communication such a challenge for healthcare professionals.

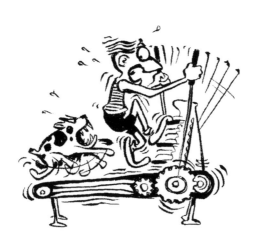

Even exercise can cause unexpected risks.

6

WHAT PATIENTS DON'T KNOW ABOUT RISKS

Life is a sexually transmitted, terminal disease.

Everyone's life is a journey through thousands of risks. They come in all shapes and sizes. Some are highly unlikely; even freaky, yet fatal. Some are more likely, but they may be less serious. Some can be influenced by what we do; some cannot. Some come from our external environment; some seemingly come from inside our bodies or our minds.

I predict that every reader will be comfortable with endorsing this easy listing of the diversity of risks. However, this too cloaks an important truth. Despite the fact that everyone feels they know what a risk is—let's define it for now as "the possibility of harm happening to ourselves or someone or something we cherish," *the reality is that most of the public has no idea of all the things that actually constitute risks.*

It is usually easy to identify the *reality of harm* in healthcare settings. On the other hand, that clarity soon becomes confusing and complicated when you move to try to define the web of potential causes of the harm – in other words, what really make up the risks.

CONTRIBUTORY FACTORS ARE ALSO RISKS

As everyone involved in reducing medical errors will know, in most cases there's a whole array of factors that have to line up to allow the possibility of harm to become reality. This concept is commonly illustrated as a series of Swiss cheese slices, each representing some risk management strategy designed to reduce the likelihood of hazards turning into harm. However because there is always the possibility of human or mechanical error, each protective layer is shown as having some holes in it. So, with several protective procedures in place at different stages of the process, if some harm threatens and gets through the gap in one Swiss cheese slice, it will almost certainly be blocked by the next.

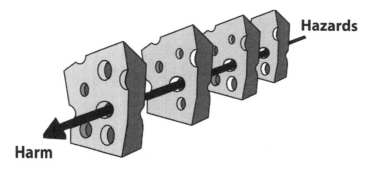

Since healthcare systems already have so many safety procedures built in to defend against bad outcomes, it is only when "all the holes in the Swiss cheese slices fall in line" that harm actually results.

This brief introduction to the many possible factors that can contribute to – or block – a bad outcome or a medical error brings up one more example of how patients and doctors view risks differently.

Ordinary citizens typically expect there to be a single cause for a particular harm. Professionals, on the other hand, recognize that there are often multiple, cascading factors involved. In all probability, if only one of these risk management factors was differently configured – one hole blocked in the Swiss cheese slice – the harm would not happen.

So, through the eyes of a professional risk communicator, the presence or absence of each of these protective factors can also contribute to the risk.

There is the risk that the surgeon's mind was partly distracted having just had an argument with someone. There's a risk that the nurse had been late getting off his shift and imperfectly wrote up some administrative detail. There is a risk that over-familiarity might lead to a momentary oversight with a sharp – or that under-familiarity might be confronted with a rare catastrophic complication.

It soon begins to look as if almost every aspect of life could be described as being a potential risk under some remote scenario.

OUT OF THE FRYING PAN ...

The important paradigm that emerges from this is that all attempts to achieve positive goals in life (including providing medical treatments) also bring with them new risks – albeit different ones, with different levels of seriousness. Professionals call these "countervailing risks" but most of us think of them as "trade-offs."

Doctors have no difficulty recognizing countervailing risks for they live in a world where an awareness of side effects is basic to their training. Patients, on the other hand, can all too easily view their treatment options as being risk-free. If they have a good measure of trust in their doctor, they may simply disregard the fact that their treatment (particularly drugs) might actually result in some "downsides."

This universality of countervailing risks is well summed up in the declaration on page 67. Though the risks mentioned there are trivial compared to the life and death nature of many medical issues, I find that these paragraphs serve as a useful reminder of one of the truths of healthcare risks: All attempts to do good might also generate unwelcome side effects.

I believe this is something that patients always ought to be reminded of – both in person but also in informed consent forms. The reasons are simple.

- Firstly, it is the truth.
- Secondly, it should alert patients not to take their own decision-making power lightly.
- Thirdly, it serves as a context to present the specific risks and benefits that need to be considered.
- Fourthly, for risk managers, it reduces the likelihood of suffering a malpractice claim.

For all these reasons – and more – doctors are advised to include some general statement about the universality of risks as they offer treatments to their patients.

SO WHAT DO DOCTORS WANT?

Doctors don't have time to fool around with the theory. What they want are practical benefits. More specifically:

1. They want simple solutions to do a better job at communicating risks for their patients.
2. They want some rationale – some realistic policy – for what it is reasonable that patients be told.
3. They'd like to feel better about how well they perform this important part of their professional life.

The following chapters offer some powerful solutions to all these points.

THE INEVITABILITY OF RISKS IN LIFE

To laugh is to risk appearing the fool.

To weep is to risk being called sentimental.

To reach out is to risk involvement,

To expose feelings is to risk showing your true self.

To place your ideas and your dreams before a crowd is to risk being called naive.

To love is to risk not being loved in return.

To live is to risk dying.

To hope is to risk despair.

And to try is to risk failure.

But risks must be taken, because the greatest risk in life is to risk nothing,

The person who risks nothing, does nothing, has nothing, is nothing and becomes nothing.

Such people may avoid suffering and sorrow, but they simply cannot learn and feel and change and grow and love and live.

Chained by things that are certain, they are slaves.

They have forfeited their freedom.

Only the person who risks is truly free.

Modified from web[1]

SECTION THREE

STRATEGIES
TO OVERCOME THE CHALLENGES

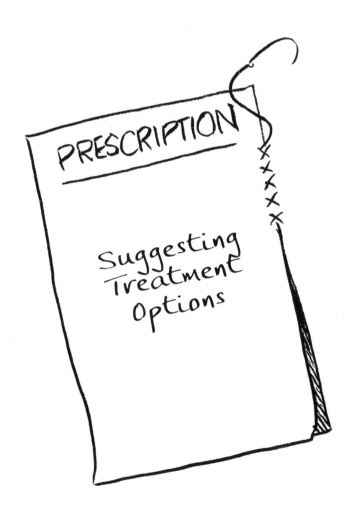

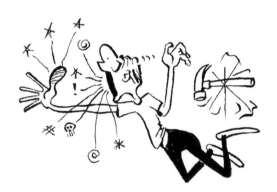

Avoid using descriptive words only.

7

FIVE IMPROVEMENTS
FOR EXPLAINING THE ODDS

Simple solutions for those who care.

W e can start out with some very good news.

Virtually all of our suggestions for improving risk communication with patients require very little, if any, extra time or money. Given the realities of doctors' busy lives, this should be a powerful incentive for them to try out some or all of our recommended "best practices."

The following suggestions bring the strength of having been tried in professional situations and answering some of the challenges that patients experience when they fail to understand risks. Not only do they work but they can also reward clinicians by increasing their satisfaction in their own professional performance.

However, having said that, I of course acknowledge that, in medicine, one size seldom fits all. This book therefore provides a tool box of strategies from which physicians can choose according to the specific needs of their patients and the particular communication challenges of their practice.

Communicating the Odds

Both doctors and their clients recognize that understanding the probabilities is a major part of the information they want to have if they are to be involved in decisions about their treatment — and also to help in planning their life ahead. In previous chapters, we identified the main difficulties that patients encounter so, with this in mind, we can now offer some simple strategies that take into account the patients' perspectives.

1. Avoid using descriptive words only

There is considerable evidence that doctors and patients often mean very different orders of magnitude by the same descriptive words. Typically they reflect the speaker's perspective and this may differ widely from that of the listener. To avoid this unintentional miscommunication, we recommend elaborating all risk communications by also adding an expression of the estimated numbers.

2. Use a standardized vocabulary of risk descriptors

This sounds like more of a burden than it is. The idea is simply to restrict the descriptive words to a limited vocabulary and to ask doctors to be more consistent in the level of likelihood that they intend by each of these terms. Since most doctors find themselves repeating the same data to different patients, it is relatively easy to sit down, list the risks and the levels of likelihood that are attached to each possibility and then chose a descriptor from a limited range of words.

For the U.S., we recommend that the descriptors on the opposite page be consistently matched to the different levels of likelihood.

This is very similar to the recommendations of Dr. Kenneth Calman in England.[1] However, different countries are likely to choose different words based upon the implied shades of meaning that already exist within their different cultures. The European Union, for example, has suggested a different standardized vocabulary: "very common," "common," "uncommon," "rare," and "very rare." Whatever words are chosen to express the different levels of likelihood, the principle is the same. Patient-focused organizations should be taking some steps to reduce the *mis*communication that commonly exists when descriptive words alone are used. Those who produce informed consent forms might also include the standardized numeric definitions of the descriptive terms they use.

Admittedly, whatever standardized terms are chosen, we should expect that they will take a little time to become established in the minds of the doctors and patients. But every little bit helps.

Verbal Description	Frequency Bands	Odds
Very High	100 – 10%	1 in 1 – 1 in 10
High	10 – 1%	1 in 10 – 1 in 100
Moderate	1 – 0.1%	1 in 100 – 1 in 1,000
Low	0.1 – 0.01%	1 in 1,000 – 1 in 10,000
Very Low	0.01 – 0.001%	1 in 10,000 – 1 in 100,000
Minimal	0.001 – 0.0001%	1 in 100,000 – 1 in 1 million
Effectively Zero	<0.0001%	1 in 1 million – 1 in 1 billion

Once doctors are made aware of the real possibilities for misunderstanding between two cultures, such as highly educated doctors and vulnerable and concerned patients, I hope they will feel sufficiently concerned to take the small amount of time necessary to try this solution.

3. Make sure you frame the odds from the positive perspective.

Now that we have clear evidence that patient choices can be completely turned around simply as a result of the *way* the odds are expressed, it is important for doctors to be alert to how they present their knowledge to patients. Obviously the doctor should always respond to the patient's concern to know the possibility of harm but it is very important indeed to also make sure that the positive framing is presented too — namely those who might be predicted to have a *good* outcome or receive the benefits *without* suffering harm.

This is such an unfamiliar practice that it may seem clumsy at first. However I consider it very important for everyone who considers him or herself to be patient-focused. The ability to exert a major influence on the patient's decision-making processes leaves physicians with a large responsibility. If that of itself were not persuasive, there is an added reason why this procedure merits adoption.

We have abundant evidence that shows that a realistic sense of hope also affects the patient's mental well being in a manner that may actually impact recovery.[2]

It is well known that an individual's thoughts, feelings and spirit can have a profound effect on their endocrine, autonomic, cardio-respiratory, gastrointestinal and immune systems in the form of the placebo effect. In some situations, this powerful process of itself can generate a significant improvement in patient recovery – so much so that those organizing clinical trials go to considerable lengths to rule out its effect.

However, those doctors who quote the patient's odds only from the negative perspective are also likely to handicap or even eradicate the possibility of any placebo effect helping to enhance recovery. *This is a serious oversight and approaches bad clinical practice.* It is antithetical to the basic tenets of the profession. By ensuring that the positive perspective is offered, there is the best chance that the patient will maintain a more optimistic focus as she embarks on treatment.

It is easy for doctors to fall into the trap of talking only about the negative dimension of the risks, for this reflects the prime mind-set of the patient. The knack is to be aware of the issue of "framing". Tell the truth, certainly; but focus on the positive aspect of the treatment – or for greater clarity, quote both.

We now have visual aids that allow doctors to show both the positive and the negative perspective at the same time. (See page 123.)

Doctors using these tools have reported a marked reduction in patient anxiety when patients are shown their positive possibilities.

4. Use frequencies expressed with a common denominator when explaining likelihoods.

Most of us are very familiar with hearing risks expressed in terms that we, unprofessionally, call "1 in —" numbers. For example: "There's a 1 in 250 chance of dying..." Or again: "About 1 in 40 patients may get this disease ..." (Technically, these are 'lowest numerator fractions'.)

This way of presenting likelihoods is so common that doctors and other healthcare professionals get sucked in to perpetuating this practice despite the fact that, as I will show, this method of talking to patients has two serious disadvantages. These are so profound that, if possible, "1 in —" numbers should be discouraged for most communications with patients and the general public.

First of all, "1 in —" numbers almost invariably are used to talk about *negative* outcomes – and we've just established that it is important that doctors make efforts to give patients the positive perspective. (Now that I've pointed this out, just pay attention to how "1 in —" numbers are actually used in healthcare. You will be surprised at how you virtually never hear the positive perspective being presented in that way.)

Secondly, most doctors don't realize that many patients will totally misinterpret which is the more likely risk when the odds are expressed in the "1 in —" format. Professional people can easily forget that in all countries there are large numbers of people who are not good with numbers either through educational or linguistic limitations. Many of these folk, under duress of their medical problems, are likely to interpret the bigger "1 in —" number as being the bigger risk. In other words, they perceive a risk of 1 in 250 as more likely than a risk of 1 in 40 simply because the first denominator is conspicuously a larger number.[3]

For this reason, we recommend that physicians try to avoid "1 in —" numbers and instead rephrase all likelihoods in terms of a constant number — "so many out of a thousand" works well for most medical risks. Thus 1 in 250 and 1 in 40 would be more widely understood if they were presented as frequencies; 4 in 1,000 compared to 50 out of 1,000. This format makes it easy for all patients to correctly identify which is the more likely of two risks. It is far preferable to expressing the odds as "1 in —" numbers with different denominators.

Notice that this simple change benefits all parties. It takes minimal time for doctors, and once the numbers are restated with a consistent denominator, they are more meaningful for patients of all educational levels. What's more, the numbers describing negative outcomes can easily be flipped or reframed, such that (using the above numbers) "996 people of a 1000" or "950 people out of 1000" will not suffer that particular bad outcome – and we hope that a good number of them will find the treatment brings positive benefits." This is a far better way to go.

Although we recommend using a baseline population of 1,000 people, some specialities like anaesthesia might find it more helpful to use "so many out of 100,000" as the common denominator for all the risks they discuss. What matters here is to establish a strong preference for using a consistent denominator when explaining risks to patients.

I concede that "1 in —" numbers are never going to go away and that talking in terms of frequencies can be very clumsy in some circumstances. However, by making small adjustments and trying to using frequencies to explain their data whenever possible, doctors can be more patient-focused. This approach has the added benefit of being optimally understood by patients of all levels of education.

5. Avoid talking relative risks with patients

Here is another simple strategy that is so important that it should be adopted by every healthcare organization that professes to be patient-focused. Ban relative risks from all discussions with patients and the public. Similarly, ban unexplained statements of percentage improvements. The need for this policy should be abundantly clear.

Virtually no one will know what the baseline risk level is for any particular case so most patients can have no context with which to understand statements about what level of improvement (or, when the tables turn, increased harm) a percentage change really means. *Relative risks cause miscommunication for patients.* For years, experts in communication have been critical of the confusion that relative risks cause – but the practice still persists almost unchecked.[4]

Taking an actual example, it could be claimed that there is a 39% increased risk of post-menopausal women getting breast cancer as a result of their taking hormone therapy. In reality, this is based on a background event rate predicting 3 women out of 1000 will get breast cancer, on an annual basis, even if they do not take hormone therapy. This is then compared with research results suggesting that 3.8 women out of 1000 who take hormone therapy will get breast cancer. (In other words, the statistical risk of cancer being caused by the treatment amounts to fewer than one person out of 1000. Over a five-year period, this means that 4 women out of 1000 would be expected to get breast cancer as a result of hormone therapy. This reality is a far cry from the public's perception of a headline proclaiming "Hormone therapy causes a 39% increased risk of breast cancer."

Instead of misleading the vast majority of patients who have no understanding of the baseline numbers, I recommend that healthcare professionals should always try to express relative risks or percentage improvements as absolute numbers. Only then will the public not be misled but, instead, be getting data in a meaningful context.

In addition, I should point out that professionals can also be mislead by statements of relative risks. For example the willingness of health purchasers to fund screening is massively influenced by the way the data about effectiveness is presented: An option offering a 30% reduction in relative risks was more likely to be funded than the identical scenario described in terms of absolute risk reduction or numbers needed to screen to avert one death.[5] Similarly there is abundant evidence that the way that the results of controlled trials are expressed also has a significant effect on physicians' willingness to prescribe different drugs and patients' willingness to agree to therapy.[6]

Statements of relative risk reduction always win the day and stand out as the most persuasive way to recruit supporters to a medical option. The reason is obvious of course. It is well known that expressions of relative risks distort the perception of the truth by exaggerating absolute differences. For that reason, it is unrealistic to expect businesses to lead the way toward change.

The responsibility to encourage a more patient-focused, transparent style of communicating results must fall on the health agencies. They, after all, have a fundamental responsibility to act in the public's interest and explain key medical issues in a manner that does not mislead. Yet despite this, our major agencies (like the U.S. FDA and similar organizations in other countries) persist in reporting in terms of relative risks, thus ignoring the fact that the practice has been widely condemned by risk communication researchers over many years.

In this way, I believe that our agencies sometimes obstruct clear healthcare communication throughout society. If the agencies themselves set an example, they would actively influence businesses to report results in terms of absolute risk figures. And this in its turn would make it easier for doctors to explain the truth about risks to their patients.

As it is, I have to admit that it is sometimes hard for doctors to follow my advice and avoid talking in terms of relative risks. So widespread is the practice throughout healthcare that it is often very difficult even for doctors to actually get back to the original absolute numbers. Not only the popular press but also most medical pamphlets communicate exclusively in relative risks.[7]

Expressions of relative risk have now become so abundant in healthcare that it is often difficult if not impossible for a patient (or a doctor) to find out the absolute numbers behind the medical reports.

I know of a least one drug company whose marketing materials are expressed in terms of relative risks yet has been doing it this way for so long that they can no longer locate the original hard numbers upon which the claims are made!

Even in reports of high profile medical scares, everything is expressed in terms of relative risks. The public is simply not presented with objective data in context so that they might have any real understanding of the seriousness of the issues. Recently, (mid 2005), there was a massive flurry of activity about the risks from Vioxx, and Celebrex yet, despite all the media coverage, I saw no reports showing the absolute numbers. Without that crucial data, most citizens will never have the chance to get a realistic account of the true likelihood of an adverse event happening to them. Even I could not get access to the information by contacting the manufacturers. I only came to see the absolute numbers as a result of Hochauser sleuthing on a congressional committee meeting.[8]

Unquestionably, there is a strong case to be made that using relative risks does not provide "information" (data presented in a meaningful context) for patients. I will continue to urge health agencies to take a leadership responsibility in this and to discontinue perpetuating such well documented *mis*communication to patients.

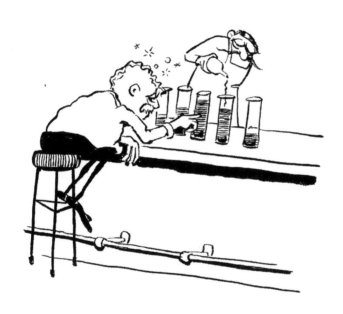

*Dr. Richard Powell appears to be the first person
to use a bar chart.*

8

THE MAGIC OF VISUAL AIDS

Putting risks into perspective.

Iff you want to be convinced of the power of simple visual aids to communicate numbers, you only have to flip through today's newspapers. Everywhere in the world, you find that when professional writers want to show the public the significance of numbers, they turn to simple graphs, pie charts, bar charts and the like. Because these familiar communications tools offer such a wide variety of benefits, it's surprising that, until now, very little has been done to design comparable visual aids to help doctors explain the numbers associated with risks.

Just think about it for a minute. Pie charts and graphs are:

- Very simple to understand after only a brief examination.
- Universally applicable no matter what topic the numbers relate to. (They are as likely to appear in a worthy medical journal as a mass circulation newspaper.)
- Understood by people from all walks of life.
  (They communicate effectively with specialists as well as people who may have less education or whose native language is different from that of the doctor.)

- Excellent for giving context and showing changes or illustrating the meaning of numbers.

A MATERNITY WARD FOR VISUAL AIDS

Doctors are often surprised to learn that most of these valuable tools for understanding numbers originated directly or indirectly in the healthcare arena.

The first pie chart was devised by that famous British nurse, Florence Nightingale.[1] She originally called it "a polar area diagram" and used it to dramatize the fact that, in the Crimean War, more people were dying from dysentery than from all the war wounds combined. It became a powerful tool in her campaign to get the British government and the healthcare leaders of that time to recognize the need to fight against the unsanitary conditions that were prevalent in her day.

The first bar chart or histogram in medicine was designed in 1810 by Dr. Richard Powell in London.[2] Oddly enough, he set out to demonstrate that, after King George III declared himself to be mad, it became fashionable for others to declare themselves to be mad as well! Although his numbers were small, he found that this trend could be displayed when he grouped them into five-year periods.

The first two-dimensional graph is reported to have been conceived much earlier by the natural philosopher Descartes as he lay on his sick bed. Supposedly, he mentally plotted the movements of a fly when viewed against the height and width of his bedroom wall. This two dimensional framework for plotting points was extended into mapping with the so-called Cartesian Coordinates.[3]

What all these communication tools have in common is this: They provide simple ways to help people visualize the relationships between numbers so they can more easily understand what the facts show.

When you think about it, this is exactly what healthcare professionals need in order to communicate probabilities. This realization has lead to several studies on the value of decision aids in promoting patient choice.[4]

TWO VISUAL AIDS FOR RISK COMMUNICATORS

The next three chapters introduce healthcare professionals to two simple communication tools that have been specifically designed to help explain the odds of different outcomes to patients. Like their better known cousins, they are intuitively simple to understand and can be applied to a wide range of specific topics.

The first is the Paling Perspective Scale©, a "Richter Scale for Risks." It allows clinicians and patients to look at the same scale together and partner as they put different risks and choices into perspective. This scale fits into the tradition of the graphs, bar charts and pie charts that have now become a part of everyone's daily life. This decision aid is particularly suitable for displaying low, very low and minimal risks. It also lends itself to putting new or unfamiliar risks into context by allowing them to be placed alongside other, more familiar risks on a common framework.

The second tool is the Paling Palette©. Typically, this is an array of 1000 simple-to-count icons representing individual people. This exceptionally effective tool makes it simple for clinicians to show – on a single sheet – both the estimated number of people who are likely to be affected by any given risk and, at the same time, the numbers that probably will not. This tool is most helpful in healthcare when dealing with risks that might be classified as very high, high or moderate – as well as those many risks that have a low likelihood.

These visual aids have great potential for helping patients understand risks across all the different specialties of healthcare.

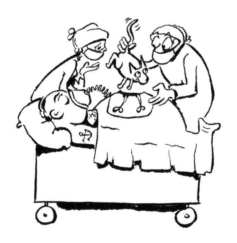

His wife said it felt
about the size of a small dog.

9

A FRAMEWORK TO COMPARE RISKS

Contrasting the worry of the week with the molecule of the moment.

You can see a simple outline of the current version of our most commonly used perspective scale in figure 1.

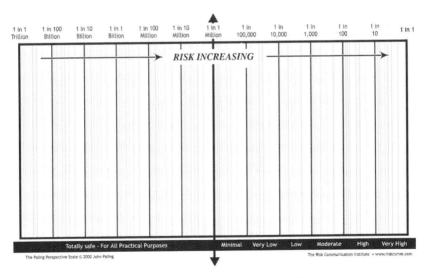

| 1 in 1 Trillion | 1 in 100 Billion | 1 in 10 Billion | 1 in 1 Billion | 1 in 100 Million | 1 in 10 Million | 1 in 1 Million | 1 in 100,000 | 1 in 10,000 | 1 in 1,000 | 1 in 100 | 1 in 10 | 1 in 1 |

RISK INCREASING

| Totally safe - For All Practical Purposes | Minimal | Very Low | Low | Moderate | High | Very High |

The Paling Perspective Scale © 2000 John Paling

The Risk Communication Institute • www.riskcomm.com

Figure 1: The Basic Perspective Scale
(See page 103 for larger version).

In summary, the design is a horizontal framework with different levels of probability displayed across its width. It allows the odds of all manner of risks to be displayed according to their estimated likelihoods. It also allows the public to visually compare the likelihood of different risks.

Before explaining how to put your own risk numbers on the scale, it helps to know something of the background of its development in order to understand why, despite the fact that it is logarithmic, it is particularly appropriate for risk communication purposes. At the same time, we need to explain some caveats about its use.

AN AWARENESS OF THE PROBLEM

My own introduction to the challenges of effective risk communication came about when I started to work with the U.S. Environmental Protection Agency. They had become keenly aware that the issues the public were worrying over were totally different from those that their experts knew were far bigger risks, based on factual evidence. They had found that other agencies were also aware of the same disconnect, and so they had begun to focus on what obstacles the public had in understanding and comparing the whole field of risks (environmental, chemical, electromagnetic, nuclear, food and water). Here are the two key issues they had identified.

1. Each industry measures risks in totally different and incompatible technical units.

2. Citizens will never be able to understand the level of risk of some new, unfamiliar risk unless they have a way of putting it into perspective alongside risks they are familiar with.

Confronted with these challenges, I approached the task as a former television producer whose goal was to effectively inform the public: I listened to how non-technical people approach risks. They learn about them progressively. Their first thought usually is, "What's the worry?" And then secondly, they ask, "How likely is it to happen to me or my family in any one year (or event, or lifetime)?" That became my starting point for my first book in this field[1].

THE ORIGINS OF THE PERSPECTIVE SCALE

As before, once you define the main obstacles to public understanding, the solutions are pretty obvious. We committed to the strategy of talking to the public in its own terms (in healthcare, that should be part of patient-focused medicine).

First, we settled on a single key unit to express the likelihoods of all the different risks, immaterial of all the different technical units that the experts used. In essence, we transposed all the different risk estimates into the one unit that makes the most sense to the public — "What are the odds of this risk happening to me?"

Second, we changed the scientific style of expressing numbers into citizen-friendly terms. For example, a risk of 3.5×10^{-4} was turned into "a probability of about 1 in 2,800.

Third, following my instincts from my previous careers, I built a visual aid to show the different likelihoods of the different sorts of risks using our citizen-friendly way of expressing the numbers.

Since I knew of no existing visual framework to display a wide variety of probabilities, I sat down and doodled with possible solutions. I soon came to the realization that if I wanted to show on one scale all possible odds from absolute certainty (1 in 1) to the minimal zone of likelihood (down to 1 in a million,) then I had a problem.

I could easily divide up the baseline into the equal spaces but, for all practical purposes, this made it impossible to distinguish between those levels of likelihood that the public would be most concerned about. (See Fig 2). With this layout, you cannot see the difference between risks of 1 in 10 and 1 in 1000. Yet these are obviously very significant differences for patients or members of the public.

This limitation became more evident when I realized that many environmental risks (and, incidentally, most small risks in life) occur at odds of between 1 in a million and 1 in a trillion. To show these, we would need to stretch the scale even further. In short, a simple linear scale was not practical.

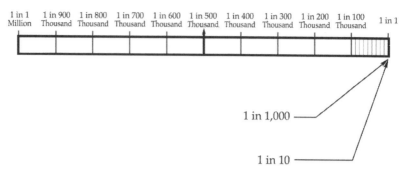

Figure 2: An attempt to show a wide range of odds on a linear scale. Important differences are not distinguishable.

My solution was to space the lines on the scale as in Fig 3.

In technical terms, this is obviously a logarithmic scale and I readily admit that this arrangement is something the public is not likely to be very familiar with. In spite of this, this design has many advantages to it, including the fact that if the scale is used for comparative purposes, then the public can see which are the more likely risks over any range of odds between 1 in 1 and 1 in 1,000,000,000,000. It also distinguishes clearly between that most important range of risks for the public – those between 1 in 10 and 1 in 1000.

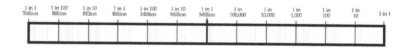

Figure 3: A practical solution to displaying a wide range of odds

In other words it is an ideal tool to distinguish differences and to see the relationship between different options. For this reason alone the logarithmic foundations of the Paling Perspective Scale© serve our communications needs very well.

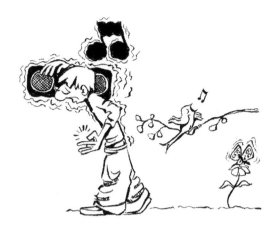

*From the flutter of a butterfly's wing to
the thunder from a boom box.*

OUR SCALE PARALLELS THE WAY THAT HUMAN SENSE ORGANS WORK

There is a fascinating physiological side bar to all this. Having designed our scale with the sole intent of making it as practical for users as possible, I found out that most (if not all) of our human senses are also based on similar logarithmic or ratio scales of sensitivity.[2]

Take our sense of hearing for example. Three noises that are actually 10, 100, or 1000 times different in real magnitude are perceived by the ear to be evenly spaced in loudness. This logarithmic way of functioning is reflected in the very word chosen as a measure of volume: "decibel."

This way of operating allows our sense organs to be both sensitive and discerning at low stimulus levels, but also to have a wide acceptance range including very high stimulus levels. That is why, in very quiet conditions, you might hear a pin drop – or the fluttering of a butterfly's wings. Yet in other conditions, the human ear can also appreciate (that may not be the best word) the output from a "boom box" radio at full blast.

This range of operational service is exactly what is useful about the Paling Perspective Scale© as well.

COMPARING RISKS

The Richter Scale for Risks is ideal for comparing the odds of different types of risks. For example, you can easily display medical risks alongside societal risks, an ability that is very seductive to doctors. Indeed, the first time that a major publication reported on my Perspective Scale[3], I was subsequently besieged by inquires from healthcare professionals from all different specialties who wanted to adapt it for their own practices.

This seemed to suggest two important facts. First, that many doctors had been looking for a way to help their patients better understand risks. Second, they intuitively sensed the value of presenting some unfamiliar healthcare risk in the context of familiar risks to which their patients could relate.

The most common example of this is when doctors compare some specific medical risk to the risk that the patient endured in driving to and from the clinic. This is usually expressed in intentionally reassuring terms such as, "You have a bigger risk from just driving here today."[4] (Actually this turns out not to be true, at least based on figures from USA.[5] Assuming a round-trip journey of 50 miles, the risk of being injured is 1 in 24,000 and the risk of dying is 1 in 1.3 million. Both of these are lower likelihoods than most doctors anticipate.)

Alternatively, other doctors try to "anchor" an understanding of an unfamiliar risk to the odds of winning the lottery or, giving birth to twins. If they work in Las Vegas and have been impressed by an imaginative math teacher in their past, they might equate the likelihood to shaking a six twice in two throws of the dice.

I support this mind-set of attempting to relate an unfamiliar risk to other risks that *are* familiar to the patient. If you do this, however, you have to be careful. Because many experts criticize the whole approach to comparing risks, I need to spell out some caveats to assist you in clarifying comparative risks for your patients.

First though, let me reinforce why I believe that comparing risks is helpful to patients and adds to their understanding.

I start with the fact that we have recently come to recognize that the way the human brain works is by comparing some stimulus *to other stimuli* – not by registering that stimulus against some absolute scale of magnitude. A person's perception of the relative strength of sensory information – and of feelings such as pain and possibly fear – seems to be related to some previous experience. In other words, our physiology works by *comparing* stimuli so it is natural that we intuitively seek understanding by comparing risks too.[1]

This important realization strongly reinforces the value of a perspective scale that permits viewers to compare some new risk with other risks they can relate to in their own lives.

This reinforces the long standing lesson taught to journalists from years of practical experience. To a newspaper reporter for a popular paper, something weighing about 40 pounds is likely to be tagged as "About the weight of a small dog." Similarly something measuring 350 feet in length translates to "a bit longer than a football field." Journalists are trained to relate something unfamiliar to something familiar and this principle is just as valuable when it can be applied to healthcare risks as well.

COMPARING APPLES WITH APPLES

The Paling Perspective Scale© works particularly well when used to compare risks of the same type where one variable can make a significant difference to the likely outcome. A good example of this is Fig 4 which shows the different likelihoods that mothers of different ages may be carrying a fetus with Down syndrome.

Just looking at this scale illustrates two important points. First, the well known fact that a risk increases rapidly with age. Secondly, it also shows the less known fact that some risk exists for mothers of all ages, not just for those over the age of 30 years when testing is normally recommended. (There are sound medical reasons for not testing at earlier years.)

When used to compare "apples with apples," the perspective scale undoubtedly has great value. It has immediate visual clarity and shows the relative likelihoods of different but comparable scenarios. In that way alone, it brings the big advantage of communicating context as well as just the raw numbers.

For a similar reason, my colleague Dr. Parker Small chose to use a perspective scale in reporting on his research explaining smallpox risks under different scenarios. (See Fig. 5.) This is one of a series of four scenarios and has been archived on our website. In addition, however, he also chose to include two other points showing the likelihood of two societal risks in the belief that they would help add further perspective for his intended audience. This brings us to confront the issue of comparing different types of risks, an issue that, in the past, has been controversial.

CAVEATS: COMPARING APPLES WITH ORANGES

The practice of comparing risks of different types—comparing "apples with oranges" — has been widely criticized on the grounds that, if carelessly done, it could be massively misleading. For example, it would be clearly wrong to compare an annual risk of one thing with a *lifetime* risk of another. (The latter would be many times greater, of course.)

Similarly, you would not compare the risk of dying from a side effect of a transplant operation with, say, the risk of dying from eating a peanut butter sandwich every day for 30 years (or whatever atypical example might be chosen by critics to parody the comparison of risks.) First and foremost, such a comparison would immediately anger and insult patients. The emotional outrage that such a silly comparison would generate would override any chance of the patient being helped by making such a comparison.

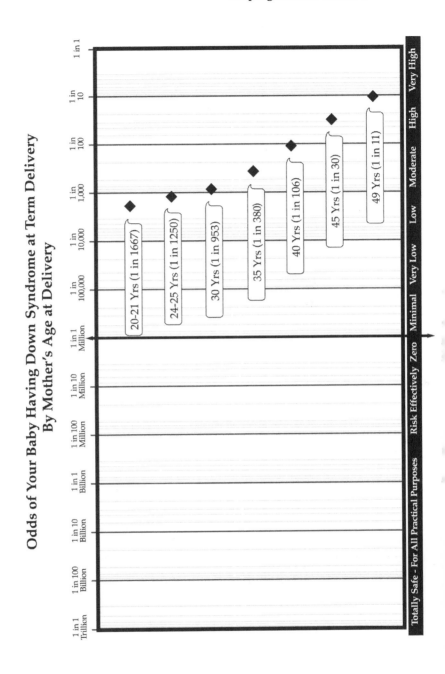

Figure 4: Full width scale demonstrating risks of having a child with Down syndrome.

However, to further demonstrate the inappropriateness of such comparisons, you could identify other reasons. For example, the first is an *involuntary* risk and the estimates of the outcome are based on a foundation of direct experience involving human patients. In contrast, the second is *voluntary* and is based on tests on rodents and therefore comes with a far lower level of certainty when applied to humans.

In similar ways, critics can claim that whatever societal risk you choose for a comparison with medical risks, it is likely to be associated with different conditions, circumstances and — most important — different panic buttons (see page 39) that will bias the patient's emotional response.

In theory, the critics may well be correct. I believe that this academic concern, however, has to be balanced against the practical value that patients receive from a comparison that may not be perfect, yet "gives them a feel" for the levels of likelihood involved.

Healthcare professionals are, above all, eminently practical people. To be successful, they have to start out with how things really are. The truth is that every one of us makes decisions about what job to take, whom to marry, when to move, how much money to risk – all based on comparing totally different types of risks. That's the way life is.

In any case, the "don't compare dissimilar risks" critics are already too late. When you think about it, the practice is already institutionalized in healthcare. All countries that accept the concept of having a threshold level of minimal risks for requiring informed consent are already grading or comparing all different types of medical risks against some practical yardstick.

Secondly, recent ideas (the so-called fuzzy-trace theory) about the mechanism of decision making suggests that where possible, reasoning operates by extracting the gist of the information qualitatively, rather than focusing on the details of the quantitative information. In other words, the brain seeks to make simple comparisons.[6]

Thirdly, doctors need to recognize that all adults already have some informed understanding of risks *by virtue of their everyday experiences*

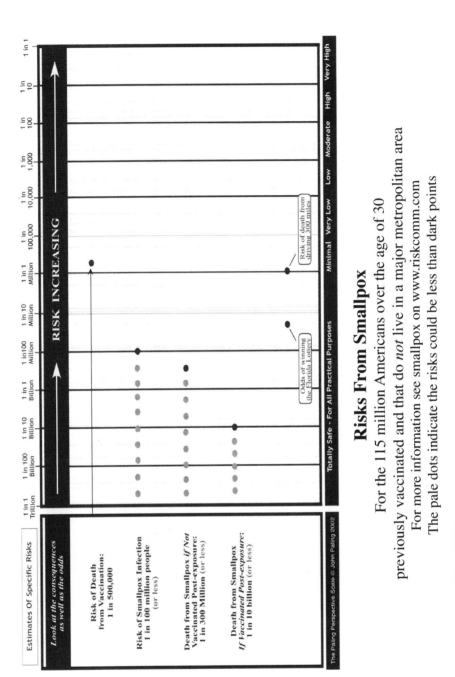

Risks From Smallpox

For the 115 million Americans over the age of 30
previously vaccinated and that do *not* live in a major metropolitan area
For more information see smallpox on www.riskcomm.com
The pale dots indicate the risks could be less than dark points

Figure 5: Smallpox risks under one possible scenario

of living. It is natural that patients should want to relate information about some new medical risk to this "unofficial expertise" when they seek their own context for their healthcare decisions.

What we recommend has the major benefit of reflecting how all humans actually think. I agree that as far as possible we should compare apples with apples. Yet I firmly believe there is great value in cautiously making "best efforts" to communicate the likelihood of some unfamiliar risks in the context of some dissimilar ones with which the patient is familiar. Here is one way to do it.

THE HOME-BASE ZONE

There is one criticism of comparing apples with oranges that I do have some sympathy for and it is as follows.

Skeptics worry that whoever chooses and defines the particular risk to be used for comparisons can always manipulate the message. This is not likely in doctor-patient communication but is certainly the case where political or financial pressures come into play. I have a simple way around this issue that actually reinforces the value of our scale in healthcare.

I advocate using not just one, but instead a *whole range of societal risks* for comparison. What's more, when it comes to concerns about industrial risks (which can take place in an angry public meeting and not in the private consulting rooms of doctors), I empower members of the public to choose which risks they want to use for comparisons. In that way, there can be no doubt that members of the public have control over what are acceptable comparisons.

The same technique can be adapted to healthcare in the following manner.

Instead of comparing an unfamiliar, medical risk with a single, carefully chosen anchor risk (that might indeed be suspect), I use the perspective scale to define something else that is very powerful and persuasive.

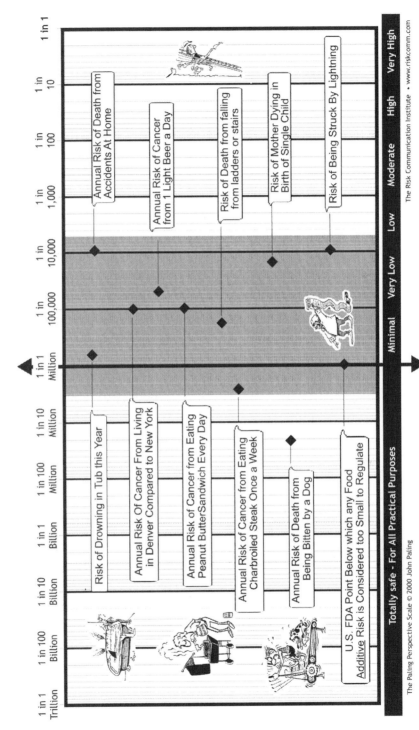

Risks With Which We Are "At Home"

The Risk Communication Institute • www.riskcomm.com

The Paling Perspective Scale © 2000 John Paling

Figure 6: A comfort zone of familiar risks

I set out to show not just one, but a broad array of risks of many types that represent the familiar life of the general public. These are easily understood risks that, by and large, all people are "at home with."

By "at home," I mean they are mainly domestic risks: but also "at home" psychologically as well. These are risks that members of the public acknowledge might potentially harm them yet, *based on their own life experience*, they consider as "acceptable" in the sense that they don't specifically alter their lives to avoid them.

When you put these together on a scale, you have a "home-base zone" of risks that can reasonably be used for comparison with any other fresh, unfamiliar risk. (See Fig. 6.)

It turns out that most (annual or per incident) risks in the home-base zone have odds ranging from 1 in 10,000 to 1 in 10 million. These are risks that, by definition, we are all "at home with."

As such, in practical terms, this zone might also be considered to define the "minimal" level of risks mandated for informed consent. (My vote would go for requiring doctors to specifically inform patients only if the risk was more likely than 1 in 10,000 – with some qualifiers.)

Knowing the location of this band of risks is very valuable for doctors and patients alike. It can serve as a useful yardstick for comparisons of all manner of risks. It isn't perfect, but it certainly is helpful when facing new risks.

I recommend that, if doctors use the scale to display medical risks, they also show the home-base zone as a valid reference zone for patients. They can explain the layout of the scale (which soon becomes unnecessary after initial familiarization) and then refer to the home-base zone along the following lines: "This area shows the likelihood of all sorts of possibly serious risks that most people are completely at home with. We consider these very low or minimal. You can now see where these medical risks we are talking about fall in relation to this."

I personally go through the process myself when faced with some new risk, and so I remain a firm advocate for using visual aids such as perspective scales to help compare risks in real-life situations.

In addition, we should add that such paperwork – indeed all visual decision aids – can be made part of the medical record.

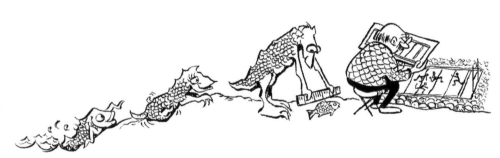

Evolution of the Paling Scale

10

THE EVOLUTION OF THE PALING PERSPECTIVE SCALE©

Adapting to the healthcare environment

The first scales we produced were influenced by the success of the universally known "Richter Scale" for earthquakes. (Another completely logarithmic scale.) That seemed a good model since it

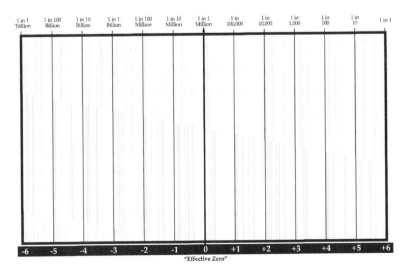

Figure 1: The basic horizontal scale with "bottom line" numbers.

clearly served the public well and was widely accepted by the media. In essence, that scale works by translating the experts' technical units into consistent, simple numbers. Despite the fact that the public does not really understand logarithmic scales, we were impressed by how, with familiarity, the public soon recognizes that, a 6 on the Richter Scale indicates a terrifyingly damaging earthquake whereas a 3 on the scale conveys a much smaller risk that would certainly shake things up yet would not cause major destruction. Hence, in the early versions of our scales, we also used "bottom line numbers" intended as a short cut for the different zones of risks. (Fig. 1, page 101.)

We designated 1 in a million being "Effectively Zero Risk" — a term I would still justify on the grounds that no government agency typically regulates any types of risks below that level of likelihood.

PALING PERSPECTIVE SCALES© FOR HEALTHCARE

After using our scales with doctors, we made changes to meet the special needs of healthcare professionals. Here are some of them.

1. Adding verbal descriptions of likelihood.

We replaced the bottom line numbers with verbal descriptors that relate to clearly defined zones of likelihood. This supports our campaign to use consistent verbal descriptors to match different levels of likelihood. (See page 73.)

2. Removing the logarithmic guidelines.

The fine lines within each block are essential for plotting the odds for risks on the scale. However, once the points are recorded, these lines can be removed so that patients are not distracted by the irregular spacings. (See Fig. 2.)

What really matters is how different likelihoods space out across the scale *so that they can be compared with each other* and thus provide better understanding.

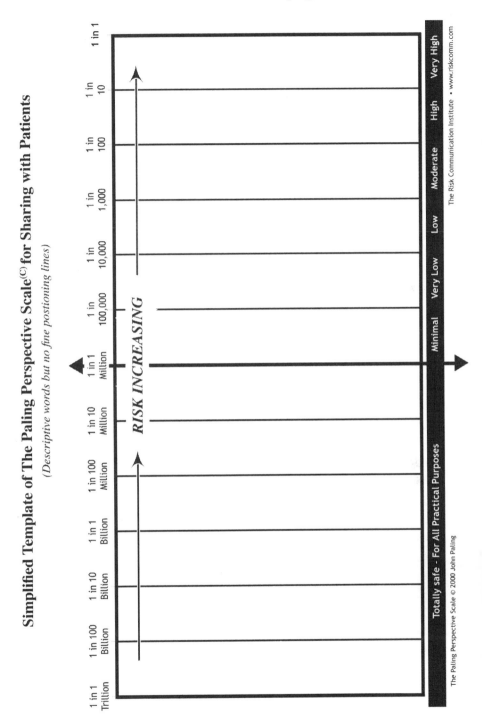

Figure 2: Basic horizontal scale with consistent descriptive terms.

3. Only showing odds greater than 1 in a million.

Since most of the healthcare risks that will be discussed with patients are far more likely to occur than chances of 1 in a million, half the original scale can be removed for most practical purposes. This allows the remainder of the scale (covering from 1 in 1, to 1 in 1 million) to be spread more widely and in this way to provide increased space between the different numbers. (See Fig. 3, page 105.)

Alternatively, you can use the space that has been freed up on the left side to show the actual numbers or the text that defines each of the points.

4. Changing the scale into a vertical format.

On several occasions, we have been asked by clients to redesign the basic scale as a vertical format.[1] (See also page 173.) On the face of it, this should work better. First, it would support the intuitive logic that the higher the risk, the higher the point falls on the scale. Second, it should more easily fit the vertical format of most publications.

On the other hand, in practice, we have found vertical formats offer less space for the descriptive text and the lines joining text to the associated points tend to be very confusing. Furthermore, they also do not adapt well to the horizontal format of most computer presentation programs such as Microsoft's PowerPoint or Apple's Keynote.

Additionally, we have many horizontal scales already in use by clients in many different professions and, for the sake of consistency, we have chosen not to use vertical formats.

Our clients are free to choose whichever formats they feel will work well in their own situations and, for those who would like to try them, we offer vertical formats on our web site — www.riskcomm.com.

COMMUNICATING INFORMATION WITH THE SCALE

For doctors, one of the main benefits of the Paling Perspective Scale© is that it makes it possible to show several risk scenarios side by side on

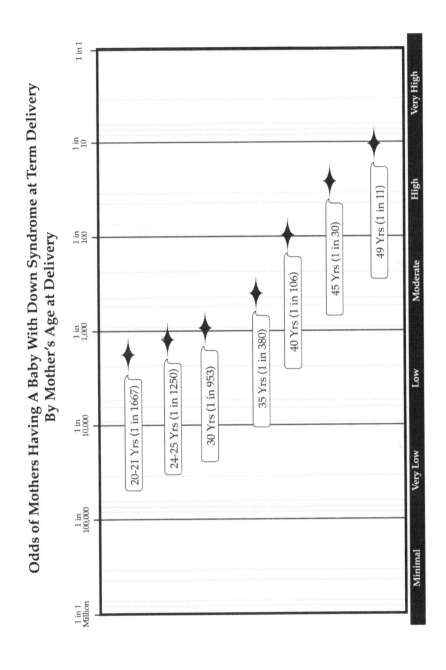

Figure 3: A "half width" horizontal scale showing how the points are positioned across the visual aid

the same document. This inevitably provides a visual context for the data that is pivotal to communicating risks. Fig. 4 from Australia is a good example of this. (See page 107.)

It is clear that the prime focus of this visual aid is on communicating medical risks, although various other societal risks have been included to help add perspective. A similar format is shown for bone marrow donors in Fig. 5, page 109.

Using the Perspective Scale can be very useful for giving a *general* understanding of the level of probability for new or unfamiliar risks. Although we accept that many risk comparisons can always be challenged on specific technical grounds, we have named a series of zones on the perspective scale to show where different types of risks fall. Each of these, in their own way, can teach us something.

We will leave the zone for medical risks for last.

Home-Base Zone

Earlier we saw the value of defining not just one, but a whole collection of "home-based risks." These reflect those many domestic situations that, under very rare circumstances, might cause death or serious harm yet, while we recognize their existence, they are not so common that people go out of their way to avoid them.

This general zone can serve as a general benchmark for comparison with all types of unfamiliar risks.

If you compile your own examples to build a Home-base Zone, (see page 97) you can't avoid this stark conclusion: *There is, in truth, no such thing as a risk-free lifestyle.* This is in marked contrast to what everyone wants to hear from doctors — namely that their risk is zero. Seen from a broad perspective, we are all exposed to hundreds, if not thousands, of risks that could result in death. However, each one has only a very low likelihood of happening. It is important for us (especially patients) to recognize that in reality, we all live, eat, drink, sleep, drive, swim, work, and play while surrounded by a cloud of potentially serious risks that would be estimated to occur less frequently than 1 chance in 10,000 in any one year.

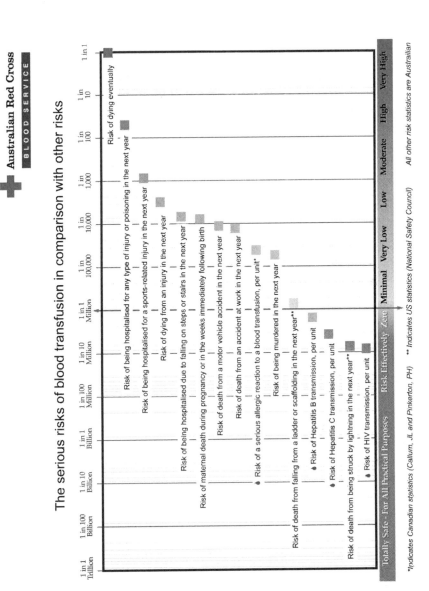

Figure 4: The visual aid customized for blood transfusion information

Created by Tessa Hillgrove and Ross Savvas
For further information about this scale, readers may contact Dr. Ross Savvas,
Australian Red Cross Blood Service, Ph: +61 8 8422 1214
301 Pirie Street, Adelaide SA 5000, Australia

By the way, this same home-base zone applies for estimates of fatalities whether you are dealing with voluntary risks or involuntary risks. As such, I consider it fair to say that any medical risk with odds less likely than 1 in 10,000 can be described as "no more likely than the risks of daily life that we all tolerate."

Pandemonium Chloride Risks

Having defined the zone of likelihood for many home-based risks, we did a similar thing for industrial risks. We found that, assuming industrial plants were operating at their regulated levels, the risk to workers and neighbors was no greater than those in the home base zone of risks. If you put them on a perspective scale, they effectively overlap.

The perception is usually quite different. People fear that if you live close to an industrial plant, drink tap water or eat foods that might have pesticide residues on them, you are more likely to be harmed than you would by cleaning house or doing yard work.

Yet the amount of concern that the public feels about industrial risks is far greater than those risks we encounter around each of our homes (where we typically feel "safe as houses"). This led me to create my tongue-in-cheek title for industrial hazards – the pandemonium chloride zone.

The relevance of all this is simply to point out that using The Paling Perspective Scale[C] allows us to give industrial risks some perspective by displaying the pandemonium chloride zone on the same scale as the home-base zone of risks.

One-Time-Only Risks

I defined this zone to bring perspective to some of the dramatic news reports that pop up in the media. People can sometimes forget that some stories become newsworthy simply because they are so highly unlikely. This becomes very clear if you show on a perspective scale where a risk would fall if it happened to only one person in the U.S. – or one person in the whole world.

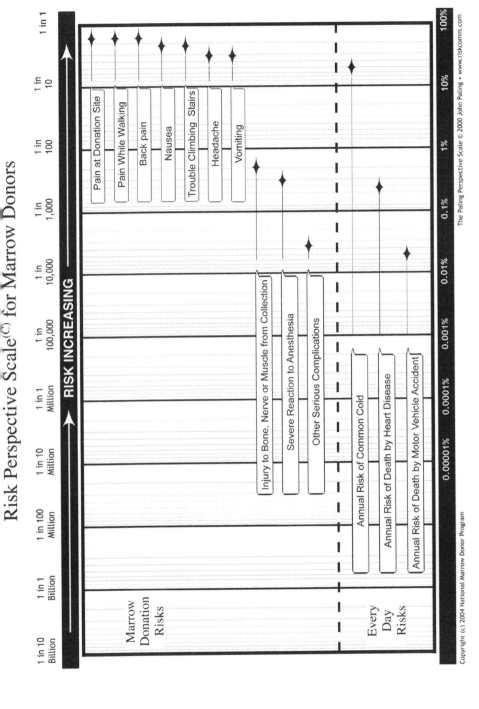

Figure 5: The visual aid customized for marrow donor information

When this one-time-only zone is shown in relation to our home-base zone (See Figure 6, page 111), it becomes clear that the events in the one-time-only zone are about 1000 times *less* likely that those risks we are "at home with."

The lesson I wanted to get across to the public was to be cautious of splashy news stories, including those raising alarm calls about risks. Before readers overreact to such stories, I suggested that they consider the likelihood and the possible consequences of the event happening to them before making any personal judgments.

Medical risks versus societal risks

Some years ago, as a member of the Department of Human and Environmental Toxicology at the University of Florida, I organized a seminar series for all those on campus who had an interest in risk assessment and risk communication. We unearthed folk from an astonishingly wide variety of disciplines. We had experts in pesticides, bridge design, industrial pollution, automobile safety, habitat loss, and risk statistics. But also we drew in the local experts on AIDS.

Most of the meetings were not memorable now, but what will stay with me was being confronted with the level of risks for contracting AIDS. The numbers were massively greater than all the chemical, environmental, nuclear, and pollution risks that we had been focusing on up to that time.

Admittedly, AIDS numbers are exceptionally high. But when you look at the world of medical risks in general, it becomes clear that the odds of most serious healthcare risks are up to 100 – 1000 to a million times MORE likely than most of the "worries of the week and the molecules of the moment" that foment the fear factors of the media on any given day.

Most of the risks that doctors talk about with patients are far more likely (and usually far more serious) than the other risks of life that most citizens worry about. In other words, patients have little or no awareness of just how enormously risky (in relative terms) their medical issues really are. For example, odds of 1 in 500 of a fatality from

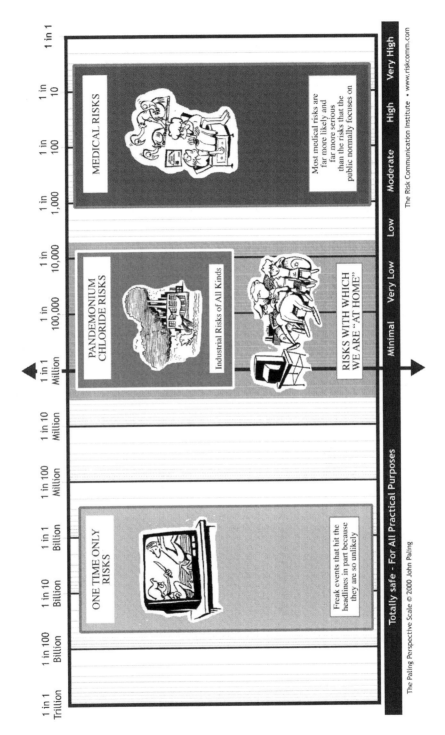

Figure 6: Major risk zones in life

some treatment is an enormous risk compared to all the thousands of potentially fatal but highly unlikely risks that the public and the media spend their time worrying about on a daily basis. Logically, once patients see medical risks in the context of other risks of life, they will become even more concerned about understanding their medical choices.

Then, presumably, more of them will want their doctors to be able to effectively communicate their knowledge about risks.

Pointing out that many illnesses and medical procedures come with such high levels of risks is not, of course, a criticism of healthcare professionals. Only a generation ago, many of today's treatments were not even known. In those days, the likelihood of a patient dying or being severely ill was far greater.

As a development from all this, we came to realize that many medical risks were so (relatively) likely that our Perspective Scales had limited value in displaying moderate, high and very high risks. For that reason we designed a totally different visual aid, the Paling Palette©, which is the topic of the next chapter.

SUMMARY:
THE BENEFITS OF
PERSPECTIVE SCALES

1. They allow low likelihood risks to be visually displayed so that patients can compare the probabilities of different outcomes or choices.

2. They have been successfully used for communicating risks to both professionals and the public in a wide variety of situations over many years..

3. They define the zone of likelihood for serious or fatal risks that citizens in general are "at home with". This can provide context for patients to view medical risks they may be confronted with.

4. They may be used to more logically define the level of risks that doctors might be expected to explain to patients as part of the informed consent process.

Readers may download high resolution versions of these perspective scales for trial purposes from www.riskcomm.com

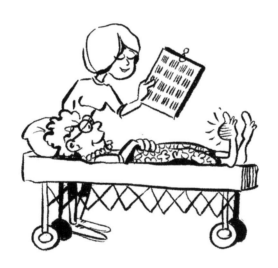

*Footnote: Visual Aids can make
the numbers easily understandable.*

11

THE POTENTIAL OF THE PALETTES

The obvious takes a little longer

Many of the risks that doctors need to address are far more likely to occur — say affecting between 1 in 1000 to 1 in 10 people — and for these, we came up with a far more appropriate communications tool, The Paling Palette©. (Fig. 1)

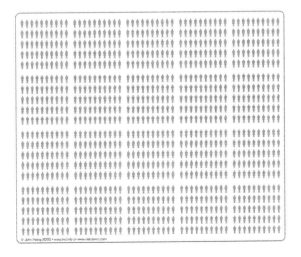

Figure 1: 1000 "little people" laid out so they can be easily counted

The concept and designs of palettes seem blindingly obvious now. Nevertheless, they were in fact developed and tested in a series of progressive improvements as we tried to adapt our perspective scales for healthcare. The resulting palette designs have been tested with patients in genetic counseling and transplant surgery scenarios but far more testing and evaluation is needed in clinical settings. For this reason, we make them easily available for testing. (See page 125.)

Happily other researchers have carried out an extensive qualitative study on different communication formats used in healthcare and, although the specific design of our palettes were not available to them when they carried out their study, it is clear that the concept behind these decision aids is strongly validated by their findings.[1, 2]

THE ESSENCE OF A PALING PALETTE[(c)]

Our palettes are so simple that a description is almost redundant. In the most commonly used version, we display a grid composed of 1000 small icons, each representing a single actual person. Upon this framework, a doctor or genetic counselor can mark the estimated number of people out of one thousand who might be expected to experience any specific unfavorable outcome.

Just as important are those little persons that are *not* marked in any way. They automatically indicate the estimated number out of a thousand that are NOT expected to encounter the unfavorable outcome.

In other words, this palette format automatically shows the positive perspective as well as the negative perspective – thus totally solving an important problem that we referred to earlier.

Another huge benefit is that no one, whatever their educational level or native language, can misunderstand risk communicated as a selected number of individuals out of 1000 pictures of recognizable little people. This is an important benefit for all patients but especially for illiterate or marginally literate people — or speakers of other languages.

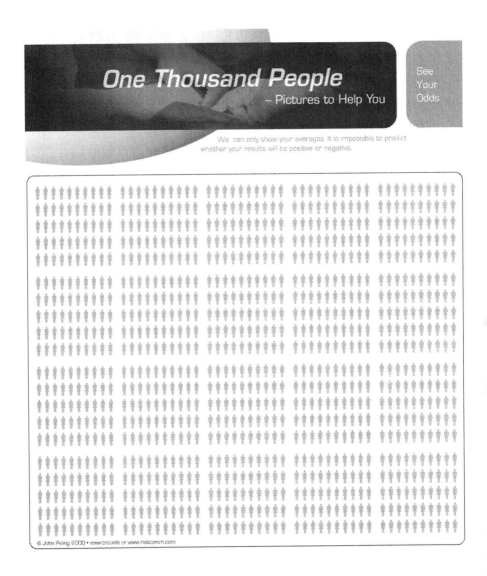

(Our design incorporates a space below the visual aid that is intended for appropriate explanatory text and contact or marketing information from the supplier)

Figure 2: A reduced copy of our Full Page "women only" Palette — ideal for genetic counselors.

The research done on the effectiveness of a wide range of visual aids in healthcare concluded:[1] "A consistent theme in our analysis was that frequency graphics using human figures were easy to identify with, were understandable, and conveyed a meaningful message. The human figures added contextural meaning to the numeric information presented because of the depiction of a person ... in the graphics."

We produce these palettes as different versions representing different populations of people: all men, all women, family (which we designate as 1 man, 1 woman, 1 boy and 1 girl, roughly randomized), all children etc. Such customized sheets can be used for doctors or genetic counselors who mainly talk to one subset of patients from the general population.

We also found that different styles of palettes were being requested for different situations. Doctors working on the wards usually prefer small-sized versions that could fit into their white coat pockets. In contrast, desk-based healthcare professionals such as genetic counselors preferred full letter-sized palettes that are more suitable for an office consultation.

As we redesigned the palettes in different sizes, we found that some configurations worked better than others. (Compare Figs. 2 and 3.) When used as letter-sized sheets, the palette works best as 5 blocks of 50 people across (and 4 blocks down) whereas for the smaller palettes, they fit better by having 4 blocks of 50 people across (and 5 blocks down).

The palettes can be preprinted to cover the most common communications needs in a particular practice or blank palettes can be filled in by the doctor as he sits side by side with the patient and illustrates the data of his communication as he talks. (A practice that we strongly encourage because of its potential to increase doctor-patient bonding.)

To make it easier for a doctor to count off the number of people estimated to be affected out of the thousand, the icons are grouped in ranks of 10 across and 5 down; 50 per group. This makes it an easy process for a doctor to accurately highlight any number on a palette.

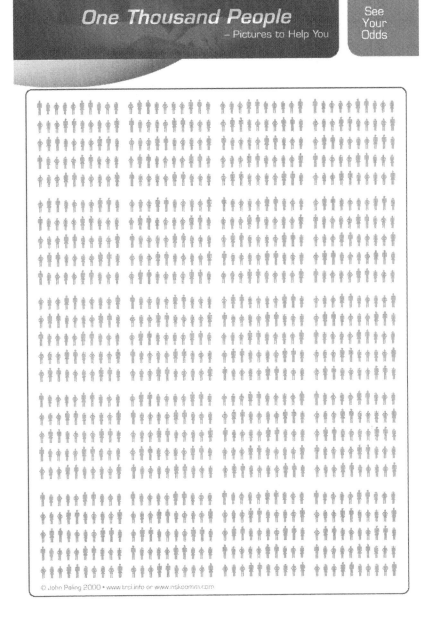

Figure 3: A Pocket-sized (narrow format) "Family" Palette comprising icons of men, women and children.

(Just imagine yourself simply counting off and marking say, 12, 27 or 283 out of the 1000 "little people" in the presence of a patient.)

Some healthcare professionals might think about randomizing the number of affected individuals across the population of people, just as they would be in life. This might mean that, instead of seeing the estimated number of affected people ranked side by side at the top of a palette, say the first 12 of the thousand icons, those marked as affected might be, say, numbers 6, 23, 103, 105, 279, 432, 480, 698, 706, 778, 854 and 913. We have already tried this approach and can report that it has serious disadvantages.

First, randomizing those icons representing affected people can be a time consuming process that makes it impracticable to do in the presence of a patient.

Secondly, randomizing the affected people makes it far harder to see the differences between two different scenarios. For example, when randomized, 57 out of 1000 and 84 out of 1000 look indistinguishable at first sight. Our experience is validated by Schapira et al.[1]

Coronary Artery Disease and The Framington Risk Factor Tables

There are several sophisticated studies in the different medical specialties that help physicians estimate the level of specific risks for individual patients. One well known one is the Framington Study,[2] which provides point ratings for different parameters that increase the risk of CAD (age, gender, blood pressure, smoking, cholesterol history etc). At first sight, such a multi-factored risk estimator may not seem compatible with our simple, unidimensional palettes. However, nothing could be further from the truth.

In fact, after the points have been aggregated based on the Framington Study, there is a conversion table that allows the point total to be translated into an estimate of the percentage risk over a ten year period. For example, a point total of 5 represents a 10-year risk of 2%. Clearly, our palettes are perfect to show this to patients as

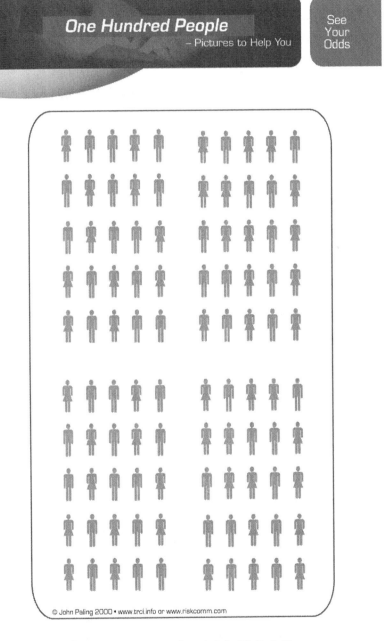

Figure 4: A Half-sized "Mixed Adult" Palette comprising 100 icons of men and women.

(Designed for medical professionals who work in areas of healthcare where risks are normally reported as percentages)

20 out of 1000 people; in other words 980 would not be expected to suffer CAD in that particular scenario. In other words, after all the complexity of getting a point total, the result can be clearly displayed on a palette.

Transplant Surgery

Another variation of our palette was produced at the request of colleagues who work with transplant patients. The normal practice here is for the odds of potential outcomes to be expressed as percentages. In order to also meet the needs of these professionals, we offer palettes that allow probabilities to be shown as the number of little people that are marked on a template background of one hundred icons. (See Fig. 3)

One of the first ways that these palettes were tested was to use them to assess whether patients understood the risk of death or, better, the likelihood of survival, over different time periods after an organ transplant. The doctor or clinical psychologist would explain the survival figures taking into account the particular patient's circumstances and then, towards the end of encounter ask, "If 100 patients with your illness [specified] and a comparable level of severity received a [heart, liver, lung, kidney] transplant today, how many of them would likely still be alive 1 year from now? Three years from now? Five years from now?"

At each point, the patient would be asked to indicate her response by marking the appropriate number of little people on 3 blank palettes. This simple procedure gives the doctor a simple test to assess whether the patient has a reasonable understanding of what she might be undertaking.

As a practical matter, if doctors use palettes in this way, it makes sense to laminate them in transparent plastic and provide the patient with an erasable color marker so that the sheets can be quickly wiped clean and reused.

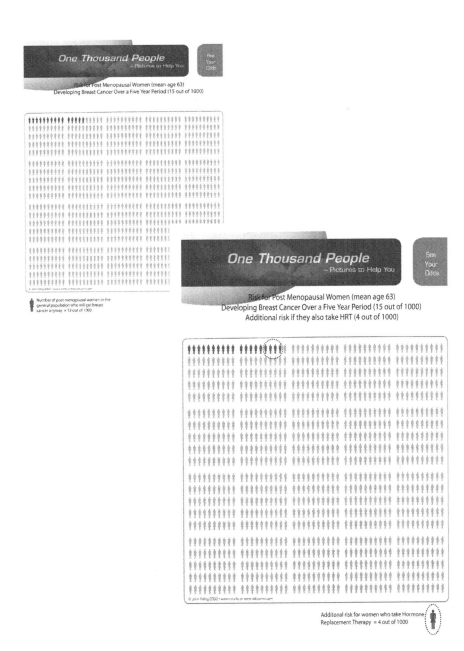

Figure 5: Two palettes that show the difference in likelihood under two defined scenarios

(By printing a series of related palettes on transparent plastic and ensuring that the upper layers correctly align over the lower ones, it is possible to demonstrate a progressive series of risks, for example, increase in risks with age of patient.)

Other Types of Palettes

We have also been asked for palettes that show 10,000 icons of little people. However these numbers are simply impractical to show clearly on a single sheet. Instead, we recommend that doctors wanting to communicate risks as a proportion of 10,000 people simply print off 10 sheets of the 1000 person palettes and clip them together and work from these.

Similarly, if someone really wanted to accurately display what the odds of one in a million looked like, they could print out and box up 1000 of the 1000 people palettes and randomly mark one individual and then invite someone to quickly find that person. This would emphasize how unlikely it would be that any individual would be affected by a 1-in-a-million risk.

Using palettes to compare risks

When physicians first learn about our palettes, they immediately recognize the benefits they offer and see how simple it would be to introduce them alongside their existing practices. Palettes are ideal when a physician just wants to communicate the absolute numbers for a single risk scenario. However in many clinical situations, the doctor wants to present more than one risk scenario in order to show the patient their choices. At first sight, this can get confusing but, with a little ingenuity, it can usually be achieved. (See Fig. 5)

Undoubtedly, the most effective (but costly) way to compare risks under similar scenarios is to print a series of related palettes on transparent plastic and then "build" progressive layers showing more and more people affected for example with increasing age. This is something that patient-focused drug companies should consider doing. A similar result can be obtained by "layering" Powerpoint (Microsoft) or Keynote (Apple) slides during computer driven presentations.

All in all, we have found that the simple 1000 person palette is an amazingly versatile tool that is ideal for showing the majority of the serious risks that must be addressed in the healthcare arena.

SUMMARY: THE BENEFITS OF PALETTES

1. They are intuitively simple to understand by people of all ages, all educational levels and different linguistic and cultural traditions.

2. They always display likelihoods as frequencies (a number out of 1000) rather than the probabilities which enables far more patients to accurately compare their choices.

3. They show the positive outcome as well as the possible negative outcomes so the patient can also be directed towards the benefits of treatment.

4. There is strong independent evidence that patients relate well to the numbers displayed as little outlines of people.

5. As discussed later, they can serve as a valuable tool to facilitate doctor-patient bonding.

6. Putting all these features together, we consider palettes to be the crown jewels of decision aids.

Readers may download high resolution versions of these perspective scales for trial purposes from www.riskcomm.com

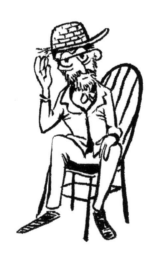

Eh?

12

CUTTING EDGE LESSONS
ABOUT CONSEQUENCES

Or, as Vincent Van Gogh said, "Eh?"

So far, we have only talked about ways to communicate likelihoods or frequencies. Now we need to address the fact that this parameter is no more than half the equation of what actually defines a risk. Returning to basics, everyone acknowledges that a big risk is some combination of a serious consequence as well as a high likelihood. This means that ideally effective risk communication should concern itself with quantifying the estimated size of both these two poles. (See Fig. 1, page 129.) Thus, we now need to address the challenges of how doctors might effectively explain the potential *consequences* of the different risks to their patients.

QUANTIFYING THE CONSEQUENCES

Summarizing the main things that might go wrong is, of course, usually easy for professionals to do. However, consequences actually have more dimensions to them than most doctors recognize.

Thomas Dalglish, Director of the Office of Research Integrity, University of Louisville, defines four vectors associated with the consequences of a risk — in addition to likelihood. These are the nature, the severity, the frequency, and the overall duration of possible harm. In an ideal world, each of these should be addressed.

Such thoroughness is usually impracticable. However, it turns out that, even where the *facts* of a potentially adverse outcome may be fully known, the *actual impact on an individual patient* may be very difficult to quantify. In some situations, a particular adverse outcome may be received very differently depending on the patient's values and expectations.

Whenever I think of this issue, I am reminded of the observations that Dr. Kenneth Kellner, Professor of OB-GYN at the University of Florida shared with me early in my work in this field. Although a very experienced doctor, he told me candidly, "I am continually astonished at the dramatically diverse responses that prospective mothers show on learning they are destined to have a child with Down syndrome. Some are grief stricken and wish to abort immediately whereas others take it as "a gift from God" and accept the newborn with love and affection. And when I attempt to predict their response, I'm more often wrong than right."

This is a prime example of how, while the *description* of the possible outcome ("a child with Down syndrome") may be objective, yet the actual *consequences* are to some degree subjective. There is no way of predicting with any precision how painful a certain treatment may be, or how different people will be psychosocially or economically affected by the removal of a leg or a breast or a lung – or being incontinent for life or being disfigured. All these outcomes sound terrifying and are clearly unwelcome but, deep down we know that some are far worse outcomes than others. Different people may respond quite differently and may experience any one of them as more or less debilitating.

Finally, death itself – the worst of all outcomes for most people – actually be may be viewed as welcome when considered against the other alternatives that may be all that remains for, say, very old or very ill patients.

The Lessons from Considering Consequences

When you add all these issues together, what it comes down to is this: Although the potential consequences of a particular risk may be easily explainable – they may never be *quantifiable in advance*.

Many doctors have never thought of it this way. They often start out believing that the common risks associated with their field are now so well documented that they can now be accurately and objectively measured and communicated to patients in an evidence-based manner.[1] On the contrary, we conclude that, because the consequences side of the equation (odds X consequences) has to remain largely descriptive, the actual size of a particular risk inevitably remains somewhat subjective too.

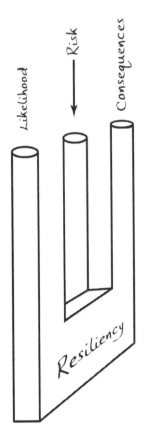

Figure 1: The actual size of a risk will always be somewhat uncertain and the consequences impossible to truly quantify.

Because of this, it is both inevitable as well as necessary that patients assess risks by viewing their knowledge of the facts through an emotional filter.

Doctors offer estimates from populations; patients seek certainties for individuals.

In this light, doctors should be respectful of the importance of patients' feelings as they wrestle to understand risks.

Risk managers and insurance professionals know that building resiliency (especially maintaining a healthy lifestyle) offers the best foundation against all types of hazards.

And it gets even more subjective when you add in the fact that, in real life circumstances, the risk needs to be balanced against the likelihood of achieving one or more benefits (also hard to quantify). Taken together, these realities show why seeking to predict an individual's risks with certainty (not just the likelihood component) may be always be an illusion.

Accepting this line of thinking brings up two important issues. First, it should reinforce healthcare professionals' tolerance for the way that patients actually assess risks. Instead of possible feelings of frustration when patients resort to their emotions when assessing medical decisions, doctors might more easily see it as inevitable and view the practice with renewed respect. Once this is accepted, it becomes part of the job of healthcare professionals to work with this reality as they strive to get across their knowledge of the odds and the consequences. (This topic is addressed in Chapter 14.)

Second, it is salutary to realize that the imprecision in *the patient's understanding* of the description of consequences of a risk can exceed any imprecision in the communication of likelihoods. Patient-focused doctors therefore should try to explain empathetically how the risks might affect patients' lives as well as simply what might go wrong.

In summary, we return to the fact that, in practice, most risk communication translates to making best efforts to *report* on the possible consequences and to *quantify* the likelihoods – and to *outline* the intended benefits.

The most important conclusion from all this may be that doctors should keep in mind that, whatever the particular healthcare issue, making decisions under conditions of such uncertainties is a psychologically difficult task for all patients.

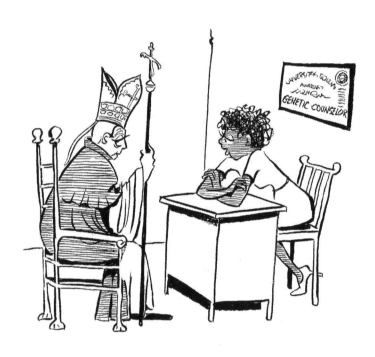

And did the virgin Mary have any sisters...
and did they have any offspring?

13

GENETIC COUNSELORS — V.I.P.S FOR RISKS

Is the Pope a Catholic?

Genetic counseling is clearly on the threshold of a massive expansion. Tests already exist for about 450 conditions and, with our ever-increasing knowledge of the human genome, genetic counselors are clearly going to be in the front ranks of risk communicators for the indefinite future.

I have come to believe that these professionals may be best placed to take advantage of the visual aids outlined in this book. Consider:

1. They are already specialists in discussing difficult risks — the possible genetic abnormalities and susceptibilities of unborn babies.
2. They already have good resources to help them understand the challenges of risk communication in their field.[1]
3. Their consultations take place in the relatively relaxed atmosphere of an office where the counselor can elaborate on the data at a level appropriate to the needs of the client.
4. The profession is currently evaluating how best to carry out its prime responsibilities of risk assessment and client education.[2]

5. Finally, if their clients really wish, they can take information away, consult with their partners and take their time to thoroughly consider the risks and the benefits before they make their choice.

In many ways, the process of helping pregnant women understand the risks and benefits of amniocentesis is (relatively speaking) fairly straightforward and so it makes a good test platform for the value of our risk communication tools. With that in mind, let us look at the process as a minor case study.

TO TEST OR NOT TO TEST? THAT IS THE QUESTION.

A genetic counselor's first meeting with a client usually includes a delicate introduction to the reality that, left to nature, about 2% of babies will be born with some serious abnormality. This confrontation with the imperfections of human reproduction is obviously the last thing that prospective mothers want to hear about. However, once they face up to this risk, they are normally open to hearing that they can accept an amniocentesis test to learn in advance whether their fetus is OK — or not.

The clear benefit from accepting the testing is that there is a 98% chance that they will be able to go through their pregnancy knowing that their baby appears to be just fine. On the other hand, if the news is bad, many mothers take the view that the sooner they know, the better.

Typically, at an early stage in the encounter, most women are interested in taking the test, but then the genetic counselor must complicate the issue by explaining that accepting an amniocentesis comes with risks of its own. Specifically about 4 or 5 women out of 1000 will have a miscarriage and lose their fetus simply as a result of taking the test. This becomes another, different risk for the mother to take into account. (Note how most real-life decisions do require us to compare things that are not alike.)

It is easy to sense the anguish that this news generates in the mind of the pregnant woman. Most likely, her baby does not have a genetic abnormality anyway but, if she tests to confirm that fact, she may lose her child as a side effect of the test. However, she also has to confront the possible outcome that may result from not getting tested at all (in this case, having a full term baby in her arms that may only then be seen to be seriously impaired.)

Confronting such healthcare decisions can start a roller coaster of emotions that have led some critics of genetic testing to claim that these discussions scare the vast majority of women — and do so unnecessarily.

And yet

Most patients want to know the available prenatal information about their babies at the earliest opportunity – whatever the consequences.

Fortunately, there is a lot that the genetic counselor can do to help the patient make an informed decision. Helping the mother explore her options is obviously appropriate. (Clearly if the mother's values would lead her to keep her baby whatever genetic handicaps it might have, then there wouldn't be any point in getting tested in the first place.)

Next, if the client still wanted to consider amniocentesis, the counselor could provide far more specific age-related data for the odds of that particular women carrying a child with Down syndrome. She might say for example, "We would expect that about 12 out of 1000 women who get pregnant at your age will have a child with that condition."

Risk communicators can use customized palettes specially printed in advance with the key figures related to that particular specialty or they can highlight on blank palettes to build up their message as they communicate their information There are benefits to both approaches but, if possible, I recommend filling in the palette templates in the presence of the patient. This has the added benefit of enriching the sense of partnership with patients.

SHOWING PATIENTS THEIR CHOICES.

Undoubtedly, one of the most important parts of every genetic counselor's job is to be an effective risk communicator. They must empathize with their clients and then clearly explain the size of the different countervailing risks. This is where our palettes can come in. (See Fig. 1, page 137.)

Imagine for example counseling a 39-year-old mother-to-be. Having delicately explained the issues, the counselor can first mark 4 out of the 1000 icons for the estimate of how many women can be predicted to have a miscarriage simply as a result of having the test. Just as important, he can flip these numbers to the positive perspective and to say something like: "In other words, you can see that 996 out of a 1000 will take the test and will be fine. Then the genetic counselor could specifically mark 12 other little people to indicate how many 39 year-old mothers out of 1000 might be expected to carry a child with Down syndrome. Again, this proportion should also be flipped by translating it to "This means that 988 out of 1000 mothers will give birth to babies without the syndrome."

It may still be difficult for the mother to make her decision. But for the genetic counselor to effectively communicate the key risk figures, it couldn't be simpler. Palettes clearly offer significant advantages for succeeding in this job.

PUTTING VISUAL AIDS TO THE TEST

Showing the risks in this way represents "best practice" for communicating likelihoods. It is intuitively obvious that these palettes can work with patients of all backgrounds. It is hard to imagine anything being simpler to use and understand, or more helpful for showing both the positive and negative perspective.

This is not just my opinion. Local genetic counselors have tested our visual aids with mothers of advanced maternal age and this was their reaction, too.

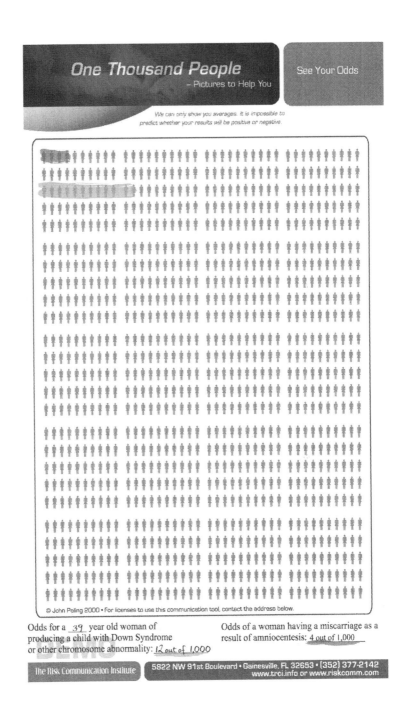

Figure 1: A palette in use for genetic counselling

In a simple test project, the genetic counselor added specially customized palettes and perspective scales to the numeric table (showing client age and likely risk level) that had been the standard way of explaining the risks until then. The pregnant women were told about the odds of incurring a miscarriage from testing and were then given their (age-related) predictions about their baby's condition explained first by words and the numeric table (e.g. "39 out of a thousand"): and then by our two communications tools, one following the other. We alternated whether the palette or the perspective was shown first and we tried to keep the time spent with each one about the same. Subsequently, the patient was asked which method most helped them in understanding their choices.

In every case (n=22) the women defined the palette with its little people as being the most helpful tool for their understanding. Each icon really does come to represent a real person – unlike the impersonal point on a perspective scale.

Long after we started to use our palettes, we found other studies (see previous chapter) that showed that icons of people leave viewers with a more accurate understanding of the numbers being presented.

One of the husbands who attended a genetic counseling session was asked if he agreed with his wife's opinion that the palette was the most effective visual aid. Memorably, he summed up his clear agreement while implying that the answer was self-evident. He responded simply with the rhetorical question. "Is the Pope a Catholic?"

I am, of course, well aware that these numbers and this protocol do not serve as valid evidence to confirm the value of our palettes. Then again, I can only keep emphasizing that one of the purposes for producing this book is to promote awareness of these tools and to encourage others to rigorously and impartially test them in their own fields. Only then will we begin to see how the numbers stack up across a variety of healthcare fields.

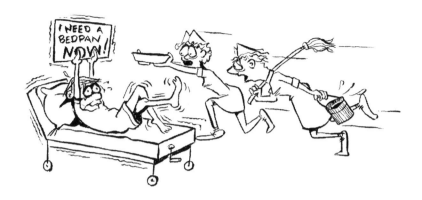

Patients prefer precise communication.

DEALING WITH IMPRECISE INFORMATION

Let's develop our genetic counseling scenario further to remind ourselves that, in some situations, it can be enormously difficult for patients to base their decisions upon the available facts — however well these are presented.

For example, consider how clients of genetic counselors might react to tests that are strongly suggestive about a potential problem in the fetus — yet are not definitive. Imagine test results coming back saying that there is a 20% chance of mental retardation or that the baby is likely to have, say, a very short life expectancy, or abnormal internal or external organs.

In these types of imprecise situations, the prospective parents often feel doubly cheated. Our new technologies can give them enough information to generate huge concerns yet rarely enough to give them conclusive diagnoses. And certainly not enough for them to easily decide about how they want their healthcare professionals to deal with the situation.

I struggle to imagine what it must be like for those once-optimistic parents who suddenly have to confront risks that can only be explained in such unquantifiable terms. It must be a nightmare. I can imagine some who might have tacitly decided to ask for an abortion had they been told with 100% certainty that they were carrying a baby with

Down syndrome now being given such well-meaning yet imprecise predictions of other, different risks. It must lead them to question what defect, if any, is serious enough to terminate a pregnancy.

As a professional risk communicator with files full of specially-designed visual aids for all manner of different risks, I often feel humbled and inadequate to help another person with how to make "the right" decision for themselves and their family. *We communication specialists can certainly suggest important improvements to aid patient understanding but a caring encounter may be almost as beneficial as any facts we communicate.* At some stage in the process, healthcare professionals can do little more than show sensitivity and provide access to other patients who have had to wrestle with similar decisions in the past.

MANY CHOICES ARE NOT SIMPLE

Research on effective risk communication in healthcare is still in its infancy and there has been little written about how best to communicate to patients when the proposed treatment can cause multiple outcomes of different magnitudes, some favorable and some unfavorable over different time horizons. Such complex situations are not uncommon in healthcare and professionals need to recall that, while we should always do our best to serve our patients' needs for information, most patients only seek to understand the gist of the different scenarios. Then they make their decision based mainly on their emotions.

This means that effective communication of the facts and the numbers is always going to be very important but that this is just one part of what the doctor can contribute to the process. Just as important is the patient's relationship with his doctor. High trust (defined as the perception of high competence and high caring) can be the major factor that allows the doctor's professional information to be "heard," understood, valued, and appropriately weighed. And that is what has often frustrated doctors in the past.

A BONUS BENEFIT OF VISUAL AIDS.

Although our risk communication tools were primarily designed to help doctors explain the risk numbers in a meaningful context, I now firmly believe that these communication tools also can serve another purpose. From what I have witnessed, when such visual tools are shared with patients, they also serve to significantly enhance doctor-patient partnerships.

In other words, these visual aids have the added potential to help doctors bond with patients in every field of healthcare where risks must be discussed.

SECTION FOUR

THE BONDING EFFECT OF VISUAL AIDS

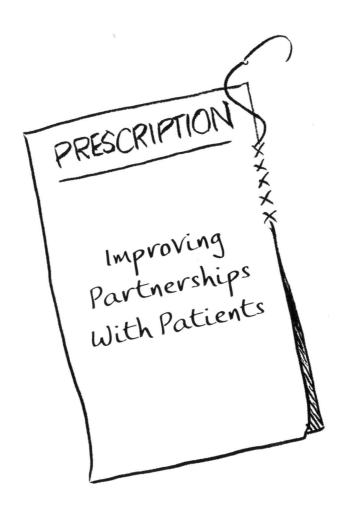

PRESCRIPTION

Improving
Partnerships
With Patients

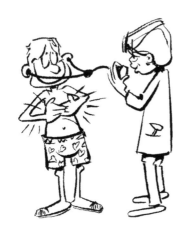

*Warm hearts win out
over cold stethoscopes.*

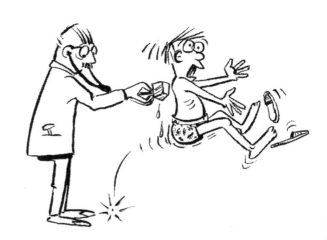

14

THE POTENTIAL FOR PARTNERING

Warm hearts win out over cold stethoscopes.

When healthcare professionals study risks, they rightly focus on understanding and communicating the numbers. In contrast, when patients view risks, emotions and feelings also come into play and sometimes override the facts. As a result, patients' preexisting notions about risks are often resistant to change. In one study,[1] about 35% of patients agreed that they had made a decision prior to genetic counseling but that decision was based on what they now recognized was a false understanding of the probabilities. Revealingly, even though the patients acknowledged that error, they wouldn't change from their initial decision. They were clearly not making their decisions on the facts.

Risks are assessed differently when they are personal. Our brains appear to be "hard wired" to consider the facts through a subjective filter of emotional expectations and judgments. Often patients don't want to know much about the numbers anyway. They may just extract the gist of any risk information to make their medical decisions. Instead of analyzing the numbers, patients are likely to seek answers to such questions as "Can this be fixed?" "When will I be better?" "Am I going to die and what is going to happen in between?"

All this suggests that we can now add "more effective risk communication" to the list of benefits that derive from having good patient relationships. What is exceptional in the case of risk communication is that the very process of using visual aids to give context to the numbers also provides a way of improving doctor-patient partnerships.

PARTNERING WITH PATIENTS

In their book *Making the Patient Your Partner*,[2] Gordon and Edwards discuss the value of patient participation in improving "the healing partnership." They offer a list of the basic elements that they consider are important for generating strong relationships with patients.

1. Patients as active participants
2. Interdependence
3. Joint decision making
4. Empowering of patients in their health
5. Two-way communication.

On a related topic but with a different focus, Dibben and Lean[3] looked at the key strategies that doctors use to build up trust as part of effective communication. They identified three of them as follows:

1. Developing shared understanding and experience. Taking a personal interest in the patient's circumstances.
2. Demonstrate willingness to cooperate with patients – especially by sharing information, trusting the patient and engaging in a reciprocal relationship.
3. Supporting the patients' sense of competence by sharing knowledge and emphasizing the equal nature of the partnership.

When you view these characteristics in the context of the way we recommend that risk communication using visual aids be carried out, you find that most, if not all, of these elements apply.

Watching patients as they have risks explained to them with the help of visual aids, I have seen how these tools involve patients as active participants. In addition, they obviously provide a focus for joint decision making and in doing so, they stimulate two way communication. Furthermore, when you recall that their prime purpose is to help empower patients in understanding their health risks, you come to recognize these simple visual aids can be exceptional devices to promote partnerships.

Their strength comes from the fact that they are personally relevant and thus highly valuable sheets of paper that the doctor and patient can talk about together. They actively encourage healthcare professionals to spend time sitting side by side with patients. They are remarkably simple yet effective. They are cheap yet deliver high value. And although they need take no extra time yet can build trusting relationships that last a lifetime.

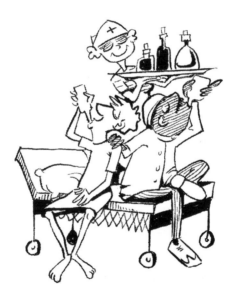

There are not many ways that doctors can appropriately bond with patients.

Seen from the perspective of all of healthcare, there are only a few ways that doctors can actively set out to strengthen their partnerships with patients. The visual aids in this book merit consideration and testing in that light, too.

VISUAL AIDS AS PART OF THE CLINICAL ENCOUNTER

We need to keep in mind that the topic of this book is just one part of the broader field of effective communication in the clinical encounter. It is important therefore to recognize that what is suggested in these pages fits well into the framework of the broader topic.

For example, the Kaiser Permanente Clinician Patient-Communication Group[3] considers that successful interactions involve four main "habits": Invest in the Beginning; Elicit the Patient's Perspective; Demonstrate Empathy; and Invest in the End.

When risk communication is viewed through the prism of their program, it is easy to see opportunities to cover all of these habits in the course of a risk communication encounter. For example, when likelihood numbers are first presented to patients, there is a clear opportunity to make a genuine statement of empathy. Something like, "I think I can understand how hard it is to put these numbers into perspective before you make your decision. So, if you like, I can show you what they look like on this visual aid..."

Similarly, a wide reaching review in JAMA[4] analyzed most of the major papers on discussing evidence with patients produced between 1966 and 2003. As a result, the authors suggested their own 5-step process for an effective clinical encounter.

1. Understand the patient's experience and expectations.
2. Build partnerships
3. Provide evidence, including uncertainties.
4. Present recommendations.
5. Check for understanding and agreement.

Once again, it is clear that the risk communication strategies and the visual aids we offer in this book serve as tools to partner with patients in exactly the way that this paper recommends.

In other words, what we are suggesting for this one aspect of doctor-patient communication can fit neatly into the framework of the broader field.

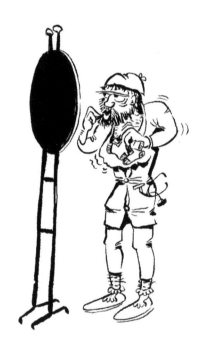

*Why can't a man be more
like a woman?*

15

PHYSICIAN GENDER & MALPRACTICE CLAIMS

Why Can't A Man Be More Like A Woman?

Risk communication is a legally mandated part of informed consent. For this reason, I was curious to research whether any particular sub-set of doctors was being disproportionately accused of inadequate risk communication. For questions like this, I like to access the extensive records of the Physicians Insurers Association of America.[1] From them I learned that "inadequate informed consent" is not even listed among the main reasons that insurance companies pay out on claims. "Failure to instruct or communicate with patient," if it shows up at all, is often thrown in later after something else has triggered the patient's misery.

However, in studying the records, I did find that there is one distinctive class of doctors who year after year do *not* get accused of medical malpractice. This remarkable group consists of female physicians from all fields of healthcare!

THE SUPERIORITY OF WOMEN

Here are the key facts:

About 6% of all malpractice cases are against women, whereas women make up about 20% of the physicians in those same areas. This discrepancy is so stark and provocative that I strongly believe we should view this as more than merely a curiosity.

In fact, I am frankly surprised that no epidemiologist seems to be posing the question in the healthcare setting that my wife often asks me at home: "Why can't a man be more like a woman?"

In most other fields of medicine, if something showed such a strong positive tendency in one of two different populations, there would be intensive studies to explore the issue and hopefully find what drives this positive outcome. But no one has. So all we can do is speculate.

Do women doctors make fewer mistakes? Do they do take less risky cases? Or is it that, in general, women are perceived to be "better doctors" in the eyes of their patients? If so, do patients who feel the caring and partnering from their doctor become much less likely to sue even after suffering distressing outcomes?

CONVENTIONAL WISDOM

When I first came across this juicy journalistic factoid, I started to ask almost every person I met what they thought the reasons for it might be. Here is a summary of what I found.

1. No one I talked to, including hundreds of doctors, was previously aware of this gender disparity in malpractice exposure.

2. On being told about this phenomenon, no one seemed surprised.

3. The vast majority of people, unprimed by me, speculated that "Women communicate better and are perceived to care more." Some developed this thought into the logic "Women develop

better relationships with their patients and, as a result, patients are not as willing to sue them if things do go wrong." (What I have since come to call the "You-don't-sue-friends-who-care-about-you" theory.)

4. Males in the general public felt exactly the same as females.

5. Doctors typically felt the same as the public – although some suggested that patients might behave differently towards woman physicians because unconsciously patients were reflecting society's traditional view of women as caregivers.

6. Risk managers in hospitals and med malpractice insurers themselves (those professionals who might be expected to know best) all supported the conventional wisdom. They felt that female physicians get sued less frequently because of their (innate?) superior ability to convey that they care – in other words the strength of their partnerships with their patients.

7. Med malpractice attorneys agreed. All of them can quote occasions when their distressed clients would only allow them to sue the institution – yet not their doctors who were clearly responsible for the error. Invariably the reason was that, despite the sad outcome, their doctor was liked and respected to a level where those emotions overrode the wish to sue the person.

Look at it this way: Bad outcomes are inextricably bound to feelings of anger, grief, suffering, wretchedness, desolation, distress, agony, and misfortune. All of these emotions can be found in the dictionary under the definition of just one word – "misery."

But misery on its own – even the most heart wrenching kind – does not invariably send patients and their families down the route toward a malpractice claim. Instead, for a patient to transition from major misery to "going after" the doctor requires a distinct decision that is, I believe, tempered by that patient's feelings about her doctor and, in particular, how caring he is perceived to be.

And, since the perception of caring is conveyed by what the clinician communicates (in its broadest sense), I suggest that we can helpfully illuminate the main causes of medical malpractice claims as follows:

$$M + PC = MPC$$

or

Misery + Poor Communication = Mal Practice Claim

Obviously a 100% success rate can never be possible because of the nature of the healthcare profession and the inevitability of death itself. This reality makes it very important for doctors to constantly recognize the high value that should always be placed on the doctor-patient partnership.

So what can we say about the gender gap in med malpractice claims? What little published research there is supports the speculation that the strength of the relationship is the all important factor. There is a clear correlation between a lack of effective communication and an increased likelihood of attracting a malpractice suit.[2] But there appear to be no studies that specifically focus on whether differences in communication styles might contribute to the gender differences that caught our attention.

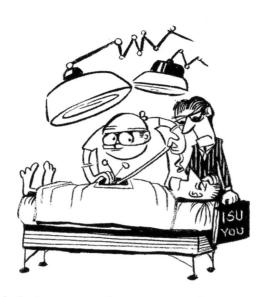

Male doctors attract disproportionately more lawsuits.

PARTNERSHIPS DEFINE THE DIFFERENCE

There are, however, several publications that report on the key differences between how the two sexes deal with patients.[3][4][5]

Men are just as good as women at communicating the biomedical facts. Meta-analysis studies show that there are "no gender differences evident in the amount, quality or manner of biomedical information-giving or social conversation." But there are differences in patient perceptions about what might be described as "female-linked communication styles."[4]

As John Gray's popular book[6] *Men are from Mars, Women are from Venus* makes clear, females operate more by consensus and collaboration while males are more independent and are quicker to seek solutions.

This reflects itself in a tendency for male doctors to feel that they should try to "fix the problem" whereas females are more likely to feel comfortable simply suggesting that they and the patients should wait until they were clearer about what might be the best thing to do.

Another result of the difference of attitude is that male doctors tend to be instructional when they offer treatments, while females are more invitational and less directive. "I want you to take these and do this…" as opposed to "Why don't we try this and see how you do with this approach?"

On the other hand, women physicians were found:

- To show more active efforts at building partnerships with their patients.
- To be more empathetic and possess a better innate ability to understand non-verbal messages (immaterial of whether their patients are males or females).
- To respond to their patients' feelings as well as disclosing their own. (In general they treat the patient's concerns in the broader context of their whole life's situation.)
- To spend longer with each patient —— about 2 minutes more on average.

Women appear to achieve strong partnerships by equalizing their status, by adopting a less dominant stance, and by such habits as inviting the patient's opinions and registering evident attentiveness to the patient's perspective.

But, secondly, *they actively enlist partnerships during the medical visit.* It is under this category of behaviors that sharing visual aids would fall; a strategy that strengthens the doctor-patient bond regardless of the doctor's gender.

WHEN MEN DO BETTER THAN WOMAN

I am clearly not recommending that male doctors should now go and ask their female colleagues to teach them how to communicate better. The truth is that many male doctors already do a superior job at relating to their patients' emotional needs anyway. We are dealing here only with generalizations.

Intuitively, women physicians tend to display patient-valued behaviors more readily than men. However, there is reason to believe that these partnership skills can be developed by anyone who has the motivation to learn. Already there is one group of male doctors which does at least as well as, and often better than the females. They are the male OB-GYN doctors in the U.S. When it comes to engaging in more emotionally focused talk, using more frequent partnership statements, and actually spending substantially more time on appointments, the men actually come out ahead of the women.[7]

It is easy to speculate on the reason for this success. Since this is one field where most women instinctively would prefer to have another woman treating them, perhaps male physicians have felt a greater pressure to learn to display the empathy and partnership-building strategies their patients yearn for. I would like to believe that building close partnerships with patients depends on how much attention the doctor, consciously or unconsciously, gives to the process.

TURNING A GRAY RESPONSIBILITY INTO A GOLDEN OPPORTUNITY

Informed consent is probably no one's favorite topic. For doctors, it tends to be viewed as an important but somewhat unsatisfactory, gloom-laden responsibility. For patients, it is always unpleasant to confront risks and uncertainties that they would rather not suffer. If risk communication were to be given a color, it would probably be gray.

The 7 strategies discussed in this book can make the process more positive for both doctors and patients. Doctors who adopt the simple strategies we bring from other professions will immediately help their patients better understand the facts they need to know. And when doctors help the process by using visual aids, their patients see the key data in a meaningful context but, just as important, they are drawn into partnerships with their doctors. The healthcare professionals can show their competence and caring at the very time when patients most need to feel that trust and reassurance.

In these ways, I hope this book contributes to a paradigm shift such that the gray responsibility of explaining risks comes to be viewed as a golden opportunity.

SECTION FIVE

TESTING THE VISUAL AIDS

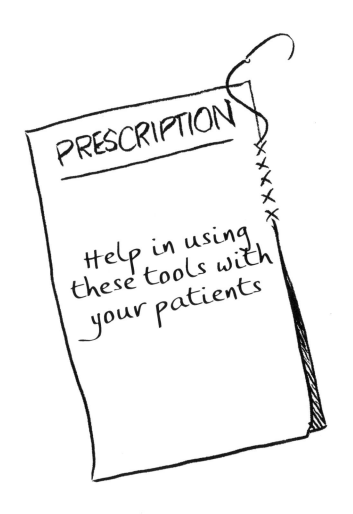

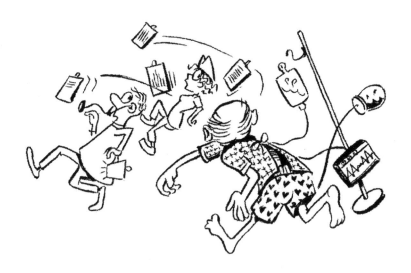

Getting patient feedback about the use of visual aids.

16

HOW TO TEST THESE VISUAL AIDS IN YOUR SPECIAL AREA OF HEALTHCARE

Welcoming Patient Feedback.

One of the two main reasons for writing this book was to encourage others to test our visual aids in different healthcare settings and then to report on their findings in the literature. We are committed to expanding the use of these visual aids to benefit patients and so we make them easily available online at www.riskcomm.com.

Purchasers of this book can register there for a free license to access and use these tools for a limited trial period. After that, there is a small registration fee to cover the cost of administering the service and to protect our copyrights. (In addition, individual licenses are offered free of charge – included as part of the speaking fee – when we deliver presentations to groups and organizations and when used as part of research projects.)

The fee has not been an obstacle in facilitating the use of these tools. Instead, we did find that some doctors encounter difficulties deciding on an experimental design when they set out to test them with their own patients. Here is a fairly typical sequence:

Senior doctors in the academic world find our visual aids immediately appealing because they see the seductive opportunity of testing these tools in their own field and "getting an easy paper out of it." Also, they see such research projects as perfect to delegate to young doctors in their team.

I think they are correct on both of those points, but I suggest there are other advantages too.

1. Relatively small projects get accepted for publication because first, there are so many specialist journals seeking innovative papers and secondly, using visual aids in risk communication is a relatively new field.[1,2,3,4]

2. Since evaluating such visual aids has not been done previously, initial research can take the form of short "test projects" to ascertain whether the topic merits more detailed studies later.

3. After a preliminary study, the researcher can explore the topic in increasing depth and sophistication leading to an ongoing series of publications in the field.

However, many doctors set out enthusiastically to test these visual aids but then find difficulty deciding precisely what to test. As a result, their good intentions evaporate. Accordingly, the notes that follow are offered as a shortcut to help potential researchers confront some of the preliminary issues before they start. In addition, in the chapter that follows, we make it easy for readers to customize our blank templates and construct their own visual aids focused on their special interests. With all this assistance, we hope that readers will be able to use their time efficiently to carry out a useful and rewarding study.

Here are three issues that should be addressed before research gets underway.

1. What are you going to test?

What do you consider "improved communication" or "improved understanding" to be and, then, how can you measure it? Here are some options and recommendations.

Are you going to test UNDERSTANDING?

In this case, are you going to test understanding objectively? If so how? Or are you going to allow patients to tell you subjectively how well they rate their own understanding? If so, how are you going to score it?

Are you going to test KNOWLEDGE of the facts?

If so, are you going to test factual accuracy of whether they can quote back to you the main risks – and /or the approximate odds of each occurring? If they get part of the answer correct and part of it wrong, how are you going to score that?

Or are you going to test SATISFACTION?

This clearly is another subjective measure but it begs the question, "satisfied about what?" One possibility might be, "Are you satisfied you've received enough information to make a decision about your medical choices?" (It might be that they had nearly made that decision before you even began to share information with them.)

2. Is funding an issue?

If so, it might benefit you to define any improvement in terms of informed consent since this is a hot button topic to sell the project for grants and, later, to publications.

In any case, it might be helpful to look at the informed consent requirements in your state or institution and see if keywords or definitions lead you toward how you might define "improved communication" in your project.

3. What experimental design to use?

To start out, investigators can use a simple protocol such as comparing the existing method of communication with the same information shown on a visual aid — with or without a pretest.

For those seeking an outline of progressively more sophisticated experimental designs, I recommend *Curriculum Development for Medical Education*.[5] The advantages and disadvantages of commonly used evaluation designs are clearly laid out there in Table 7.2, p. 80.

A QUICK WAY TO START A RESEARCH PROJECT

Ideally clinicians should decide for themselves what they want to investigate. Nevertheless, I recognize that doctors are always pressed for time so I am happy to suggest how I would approach a study on the value of visual aids (where they have not been tested before).

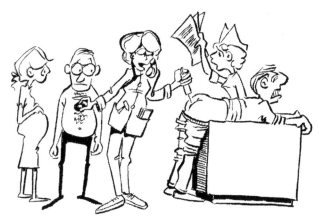

*Practicing doctors don't have much time
to plan research projects*

First, I would focus on "understanding" as the prime measure of effective communication. This is in part due to the wording of the Florida Medical Consent Law 766.103 which defines adequate informed consent as – (paraphrased) ". . . a reasonable individual would have a general *understanding* [my italics] of the procedure, the medically acceptable alternatives and the substantial risks and hazards involved in the proposed treatment..."

Then, I would start out with the simplest possible approach and expect to learn from the process (while still deriving useful results). There will be plenty of time later to make the experimental design more sophisticated and thereby make the findings more robust. Here are the two simplest scenarios along with some suggestions for questions:

LEVEL ONE - Standard approach; then use communication tool; then post test

First give them the standard information and then follow it up by expressing the information on the visual aid.

Only then explain that you are conducting a study about explaining medical options to patients

Then ask permission to ask them two simple questions about how they feel they understand their choices. (See Draft Outline for Level 1.)

DRAFT OUTLINE FOR LEVEL ONE

1. Explain the procedure and the risks in the normal way.

2. Repeat the risk data by displaying the probabilities on a visual aid.

3. Review the benefits of the proposed medical procedure. Then repeat that there are also risks. Explain that you are doing a study and ask them to please rate (out of 10) how well they feel they understand the risks.

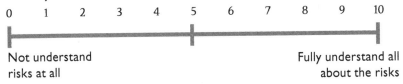

```
0    1    2    3    4    5    6    7    8    9   10
```

Not understand   Fully understand all
risks at all   about the risks

4. Then rate how much — if at all — they felt the visual aid helped them understand the level of the risks they are dealing with.

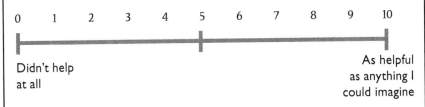

```
0    1    2    3    4    5    6    7    8    9   10
```

Didn't help   As helpful
at all   as anything I
                                                    could imagine

DRAFT OUTLINE FOR LEVEL TWO

1. Explain the procedure and the associated risks in the way you have done previously.

2. Test patient understanding: "As I have explained, nothing is totally risk-free and it is important that you understand that. So now please rate how well you feel you understand the risks associated with this treatment."

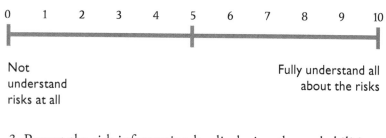

Not
understand
risks at all

Fully understand all
about the risks

3. Repeat the risk information by displaying the probabilities on a visual aid. Now ask patient to rate the level of understanding he or she now has regarding the risks associated with this treatment.

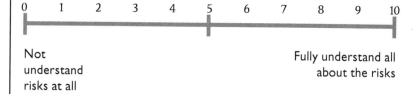

Not
understand
risks at all

Fully understand all
about the risks

4. Ask the patient to please rate how much — if at all — they felt that the visual aid helped them understand the level of the risks discussed.

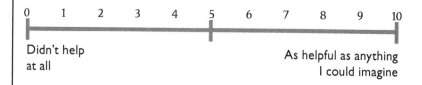

Didn't help
at all

As helpful as anything
I could imagine

LEVEL TWO - Standard approach; then pretest; add communications tool; then post test

This sequence is somewhat more complex but can demonstrate more clearly any benefits that may come from using a visual aid. Because it also demands more time from the patient (and the clinician), I recommend obtaining the patient's permission in advance for what you are to do. (If they in any way hesitate, I would give them "the works" in other words "standard plus visual aid" and not score them in the trial.)

My advice:

- Do not randomize the patients or use a control group.
- Try to include every qualified patient in the study.
- Try to spend the same overall time with each patient; if need be discuss peripheral issues.
- Keep demographic records of age, gender and time – estimates of both how much extra time it took to use the visual aid and also how long you were with the patient overall. (This may be valuable for analyzing sub-populations later.)
- Answer the three questions and invite any additional feedback.
  See Draft Outline for Level 2.

The phrasing of these survey questions can easily be improved to better match each doctor's practice and communication style. However, these two simple outlines should make it easier for anyone who is considering testing these decision aids with patients to get a quick start.

Good luck!

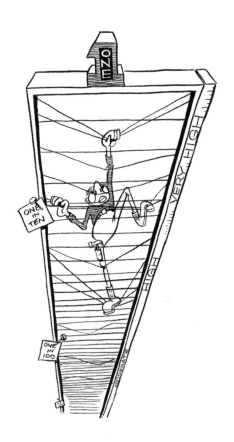

Putting points on the scale.

17

HOW TO LOCATE POINTS
ON PERSPECTIVE SCALES

It is easy when you know how.

Our palettes are so intuitively simple that their building blocks of 50 little people can easily be stacked together in a variety of ways yet they always make immediate sense. Their strength lies in the fact that they require neither an explanation for how to highlight a particular number of affected individuals nor what the meaning of the visual aid is once it is completed.

Perspective scales, on the other hand, are somewhat less intuitive. When patients are first introduced to them, they require a brief orientation session. For example, newcomers examining a typical horizontal scale have to be told which end is which. That the line on the far right represent odds of 1 in 1, or 1000 out of 1000 ——or absolute certainty. Then the other vertical markers such as 1 in 100 and 1 in a million should be pointed out as the eye moves left. In some cases, it may give added understanding to also point out where the "home-base zone" of serious risks falls on the scale.

Then, but only then, the patient can see the location on the scale of particular risks that the doctor wishes to convey.

When it comes to creating new Perspective Scales customized for particular needs, it is a good idea to try to put into the title as much common information as possible. For example, instead of starting each descriptive text associated with a "bullet point" with the words "the annual risk of...", it best to save space within the graphic and incorporate that term in the title for the whole scale.

HOW TO LOCATE POINTS ON THE SCALE

The first thing to remember is that the location of the different points is determined by the odds of different outcomes *expressed in terms of "1 in —" numbers*. So the first task is to convert probabilities that might be expressed in other units into the familiar "1 in —" numbers. Here is a quick elementary guide.

A) If you come across odds that are expressed in terms like "17 out of 3978 people are affected by ...," you simply divide both sides by the first number to get the "1 in —" equivalent. E.g. 17 / 17 =1; while 3978 / 17 = 234: Hence, the equivalent of 17 out of 3978 is 1 in 234.

B) If you start with a scientific number like "1.1×10^{-3}" (the risk of a 31 year-old mother having a child with Down Syndrome), that is the same as 1.1 divided by 1000. Hence to convert this number to simple odds, divide both sides by the same number as the top – i.e. 1.1/1.1 = 1; 1000/1.1 = 909, so the odds are 1 in 909.

Locating points on the scales

Once you have got the odds expressed in the "1 in —" format, it is a simple matter to manually position a point on the scale, along with its associated explanatory descriptive text.

For HORIZONTAL SCALES you simply have to remember that the numbers at the top extend from 1 in 1 on the far right, to 1 in a trillion on the far left as the risk decreases. So, to position a point, you must always work from the right-hand side as you position figures on the scale.

Here is an example that requires placing a point between the vertical lines on the Scale. The risk of having a child with Down syndrome for a 35-year-old woman is 1 in 378. To place this point on the scale, locate the vertical line that marks 1 in 100 at the top of the Perspective Scale, and then moving left, the first fine vertical line indicates 1 in 200, the second 1 in 300, and the third 1 in 400. The point indicating 1 in 378 should be placed to the left of the center of the space between the fine lines that represent 1 in 300 and 1 in 400.

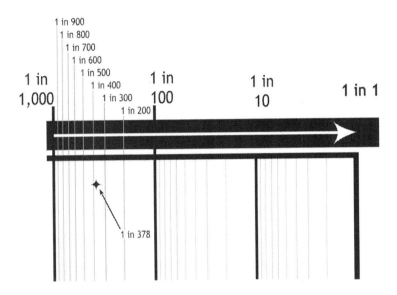

FIGURE 1: An example of the odds represented by the fine lines moving from right to left across a perspective scale

Note: This manual method of plotting points is not totally accurate because of your having to estimate by eye how far between 1 in 300 and 1 in 400 to place the point. But within the levels of accuracy of most risk assessments and subject variability of different subjects, I consider this visual placement to be adequate for general comparison with other risks. Naturally the real solution is to use a computer based program that can accurately locate the points on a log scale. We are working to incorporate that facility into our website at the time of going to press.

Also, it is obviously a simple matter to show a range of likelihoods by displaying the outlying points and drawing a laterally extended diamond marker between them or by simply showing the median point and using lines either side to show the range.

As explained previously (see page 104), we prefer to stick to horizontal perspective scales despite the fact that, at first sight, vertical formats intuitively seem more logical because the bigger the risk, the higher up the page it falls.

Accordingly, for those that need to locate points on vertical scales, you count downward from an initial marker point. For example, the estimated risk of infection with HIV from the transfusion of a unit of blood (prior to p.24 antigen testing) was approximately 1 in 500,000. To place this point on the scale, locate the horizontal line marking 1 in 100,000 at the side, and then moving downward, the first fine horizontal line is equal to 1 in 200,000, the second 1 in 300,000, and so on. The fourth fine line down equals 1 in 500,000 and the point should be placed there.

Our web site offers a range of variations of our scales including most versions in color.

The computer graphics programs that we use

We do all our graphics work in the Adobe Creative Suite of programs on Macintosh computers. In particular we build the palettes in Adobe Illustrator, and we customize our perspective scale format in Adobe InDesign. These programs are available for both Macintosh and for Windows PCs, and we can supply versions of our visual aids in virtually all possible graphics formats for both platforms. We have no association with any of the above companies other than as customers.

What stays the same

Readers who want to build their own scales or palettes should now find it easy to customize one or more of our templates to suit their own special needs. The principle remains the same – namely to display the probabilities accurately but with a context that most members of the public can understand.

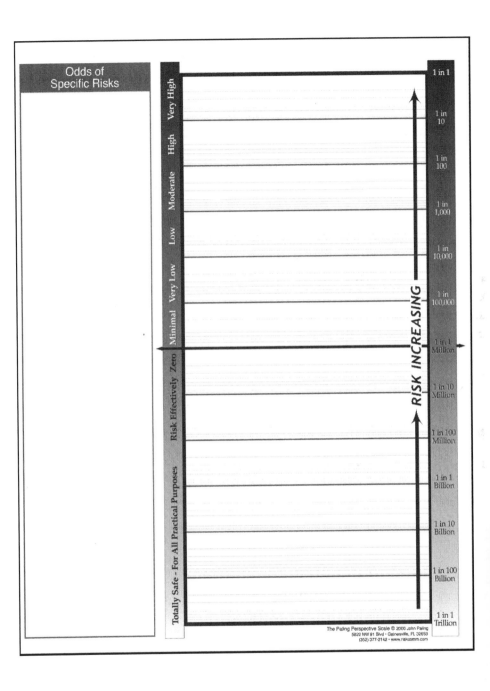

Figure 2: A vertical scale with space for descriptive text to the left of the different levels of likelihood.

173

What is also the same is that, irrespective of how good the graphics are, patients will respond to the doctor's information first by applying their emotional filter. The success of the whole process can be helped by consciously using the visual aids to also serve as a tool for bonding as well as for communicating the numbers.

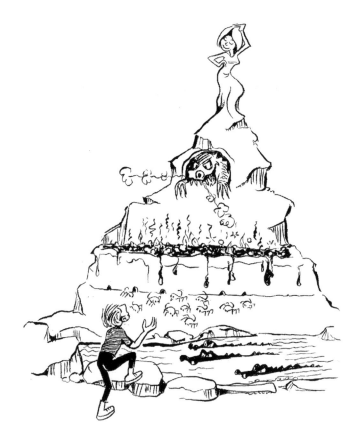

We can all be blinded to the facts when our emotional filter is telling us something else.

SUMMARY:
SEVEN SIMPLE STRATEGIES FOR
HELPING PATIENTS UNDERSTAND RISKS

In summary, healthcare professionals who want to help patients understand risks would find it beneficial to change their mindset from "explaining to..." and moving toward "P-A-R-T-N-E-R-ing with..."

P repare by first learning about the actual difficulties that patients experience in attempting to understand risks.

A ccept the challenge that patients' emotions will invariably filter the facts and cannot be ignored.

R evise the way you explain probabilities to patients. Even the most commonly-used methods can be improved with small changes.

T ry to avoid speaking to patients in terms of relative risks. Ensure you provide context so patients get "information" and not just "data."

N ever just give the negative perspective but, instead, make sure the positive perspective is always provided as well.

E xplain the risk numbers by using visual aids. These give context as well as achieving understanding for the largest number of patients.

R ealize that sharing visual aids with patients can serve to reinforce the doctor-patient bond, enhance trust and encourage acceptance of the doctor's message.

AFTERWORD

Although risk communication takes up a very small part of a physician's time, it is disproportionately important and impactful for patients. Like all human interactions, the key elements can be very variable and successfully explaining risks will never be a "one size fits all" process.

This book is full of ideas that are valuable in every doctors' "toolbox of strategies" to help patients better understand risks. They are simple to embrace. They take little or no extra time, And they stand as a challenge to every doctor or organization that thinks of itself as a patient-focused.

We invite readers to accept the challenge and try some of them out for themselves.

> *How wonderful it is that nobody need*
> *wait a single moment before starting*
> *to improve the world*
>
> *— Anne Frank*

References

About the Author

1   Paling JE, Strategies to help patients understand risks. *BMJ* 2003;327:745-8.

Simplifications

1   Bennett P. Calman K. *Risk Communication and Public Health.* 1999. Oxford University Press. ISBN 0 19 263037 7

Introduction

1   Society of Medical Decision Making. www.smdm.org – Educational Modules.

2   Elmore JG, Gigerenzer G. Benign Breast Disease – The Risks of Communicating Risk, N Eng J Med 2005; 352: 297-9.

Chapter 1

1   Kirsch IS, Jungeblut A, Jenkins L, Kolstad A. *Adult Literacy in America. A first look at the results of the National Literacy Survey.* 1993; Washington, DC. US Department of Education. http://nces.ed.gov/pubs98/condition98/c9821a01.html

2   National Institute for Literacy. *The State of Literacy in America: Estimates at the Local, State, and National Levels.* http://www.nifl.gov/reders/!intro.htm#D

3   Ende J, Kazis L, Ash A, Moskowitz MA. Measuring Patient's Desire for Autonomy: Decision making and information seeking preferences among medical patients. J *Gen Intern Med* 1989;4:23-30.

4   Gigerenzer G, Edwards A. Simple tools for understanding risks: from innumeracy to insight. *BMJ* 2003;327:741-4.

Chapter 2

1   *What Americans Say About the Nation's Medical Schools and Teaching Hospitals: report on public Opinion Research - Part II.* Association of American Medical Colleges 1998. Also www.aamc.org/newsroom/pressrel/1999/991026.htm (accessed Mar 30, 2005)

2   West DS, Wilkin NE, Bentley JP, Gilbert T, Garner DD. Understanding how patients form beliefs about pharmacists' trustworthiness using a model of belief processing. *JAPhA* 2002;42:594-601.

3   Alaszewski A, Horlick-Jones T. How can doctors communicate information about risk more effectively? *BMJ* 2003;327: 728-731.

4   Damassio, AR *Descartes' Error: Emotion Reason and the Human Brain* 1994.

5   *Risk Communication. I. National Research Council (U.S.) Committee on Risk Perception and Communication.* 1989. National Academy of Sciences Press

6   Ropeik D, Gray G. Risk! *A Practical Guide for Deciding What's really Safe and What's Really Dangerous in the World Around You.* New York: NY Houghton Mifflin, 2002.

7   *The Wall Street Journal* (Personal Journal Section Feb. 10th 2004)

8   Covey SR, *The 7 Habits of Highly Effective People.* New York. Simon & Shulster 1989.

Chapter 3

1   Delamothe T. Who killed cock robin? *BMJ* 1998;316:1757.

2   Lloyd A, Hayes P, Bell PRF, Naylor AR. The role of risk and benefit perception in informed consent for surgery. *Med Decis Making* 2001;21:141-149.

3   Broadbent E, Petrie KJ, Ellis CJ, Anderson J, Gamble G, Anderson D, and Benjamin W. Acute myocardial infarction patients have an inaccurate understanding of their risk of a future cardiac event. Unpub manuscript: Contact k.j.petrie@aukland.ac.nz

4   Thompson KM. *Risks in Perspective* volume 1999;7 Harvard Center for Risk Analysis.

5   *Ethical and Policy Issues in Research Involving Human Participants National Bioethics Advisory Commission.* Bethesda, Maryland Aug. 2001 Vol.1 Report and Recommendations ISBN 1-931022-16-X

6   Kohn LT, Corrigan JM, Donaldson M, eds. *To Err Is Human: Building a Safer Health System.* 2000. Institute of Medicine. Washington, DC: National Academy Press .

7   *BMJ* Vol:327; 27 September 2003. Special Edition of Risk.

8   Fagerlin A, Rovner D, Stableford S, Jentoff C, Wei JT, Homes-Rovner M. Patient Education Materials about the Treatment of Early-Stage Prostate Cancer: A Critical Review. *Ann intern Med* 2004; 140:721-728.

Chapter 4:

1   Merz JF, Marek J, Druzdel, Mazur DJ. Verbal Expressions of Probability in Informed Consent Litigation. *Med Decis Making* 1991: 11: 273 - 281.

2   Edwards E, Bastian H. Risk communication – making evidence part of patient choices. In: *Evidence-Based Patient Choice*. Ed: Edwards A, Elwyn G. 2001 Oxford University Press. ISBN 0-19-2631942

3   *Wall Street Journal* 2002 July 10, Page B

4   Collins, John. Dec. 2000, The Absolute Truth. *Fertil Steril* Vol 74 pages 1071–1072.

5   Sedgwick P, Hall A. Teaching medical students and doctors how to communicate risk. *BMJ* 2003; 327:694 - 695.

6   Hochhauser M, "Therapeutic Misconception" and "Recruiting Doublespeak" in the informed consent process. *IRB: Ethics and Human Research*. 2002; 24 No 1:11-12.

Chapter 5

1   www.quotelady.com attributed to "Anonymous Chicago Teacher" accessed 2/26/05.

Chapter 6

1   Calman KC. Cancer. Science and society and the communication of risk. BMJ 1996 313; 799-802.

2   Groopman J. *The Anatomy of Hope : How People Prevail in the Face of Illness* (Paperback) 2005 Random House Paperback. ISBN 0-37375775

3   Grimes DA and Snively G.R. Patients' Understanding of Medical Risks: Implications for Genetic Counseling. *Obstet Gynecol*, 1999; 93: 910- 914.

4   Malenka DJ, Baron JA, Johansen S, Wahrenberger, Ross JM. The framing effect of Relative and Absolute Risk. *J Gen Intern Med*, 1993; 8:543-548.

5   FaheyT, Griffiths S, Peters TJ. Evidence based purchasing: understanding results of clinical trials and systematic reviews. *BMJ* 1995;311:1056-1059.

6   Hux JE, Naylor CD. Communicating the Benefits of Chronic Preventive Therapy: Does the Format of Efficacy Data Determine Patients' Acceptance of Treatment? *Med Decis Making* 1995;15:152-157.

7   Slaytor EK, Ward JE. How risks of breast cancer and benefits of screening are communicated to women: analysis of 58 pamphlets. *BMJ* 1998;317:263-264.

8   Hochhauser M, Goldfarb NM. (Mis) communicating Cox-2 Clinical Trial Risks. *Journal of Clinical Research Best Practices* 2005 Vol 1; No.4 April. http://www.firstclinical.com/resources/Cox2.pdf (Accessed July 2005).

Chapter 7

1   Nightingale, Florence, 1858. *Notes on matters affecting the health, efficiency and hospital administration of the British army, founded chiefly on the experience of the late war.* London: Harrison and Sons, 1858.

2   *Bandolier 30 -1* August 1996 p.1 Evidence-based kings. http://www.jr2.ox.ac.uk/bandolier/band30/b30-1.html accessed Aug 2005.

3   www.scienceworld.wolfram.com/biography/Descartes.html Accessed 10/25/04

4   O'Connor A, Edwards A. The role of decision aids in promoting evidence-based choice. pp. 220-242. In *Evidence-based Patient Choice.* 2001 Ed: Edwards A, Elwyn G. Oxford University Press. ISBN 0-19-2631942.

Chapter 8

1   Paling JE. *Up to Your Armpits in Alligators? How to sort out what's worth worrying about.* Gainesville, FL. Risk Communication and Environmental Institute 1997.

2   Stevens, SS. *Psychophysics. Introduction to its Perceptual, Neural and Social Prospects.* 1975. pp329 John Wiley & Sons ISBN 0-471-82437-2

3   Stix G. Why worry? 1995 *Scientific American.* May.

4   Edwards A. Communicating risks through analogies. *BMJ* 2004;327:749

5   Itasca IL and National Safety Council. (2004) *Injury Facts. 2004 Edition.* ISBN 0-87912-258-7.

6   Lloyd A, Hayes P, Bell PRF, Naylor AR. The role of risk and benefit perception in informed consent for surgery. *Med Decis Making* 2001;21:141-149.

Chapter 9

1   Paling JE, Strategies to help patients understand risks. *BMJ* 2003;327:745-8.

Chapter 10

1   Schapira MM, Nattinger AB, McHorney CA. Frequency or Probability? A Qualitative Study of Risk Communication Formats Used In Health Care. *Med Decis Making* 2001;21:459-467. (Specifically p. 462.

2   Etling LS, Martin CG, Canter SB, Rosenthal EB. Influence of data display formats on physician investigators' decisions to stop clinical trials: Prospective trial with repeated measures. *BMJ* 1999;318:1527-1531.

3   Wang TJ, Massaro JM, Levy D, Vasan RS, Wolf PA, D'Agostino RB, Larson MG, Kannel WB, Benjamin EJ. A Risk Score for Predicting Stroke or Death for Individuals with New-Onset Atrial Fibrillation in the Community: The Framingham Heart Study. *JAMA* 2003;290:1049-1056. Also http://www.nhlbi.nih.gov/about/framingham/index.html (accessed Aug 2005.)

Chapter 11

1   Ghosh A Analogy in medicine: Is it evidence based? 2003.http://bmj.bmjjournals.com/cgi/eletters/327/7417/749#37190 Response to web version of Edwards A. Communicating risks through analogies. *BMJ* 2003;327:749

2   O'Connor AM, Legare F, Stacey D. Risk communication in practice: the contribution of decision aids. *BMJ* 2003;327:736-40

Chapter 12

1   Gates EA. Communicating Risk in Prenatal Genetic Testing. *JMWH* 2004;49:220-26.

2   Butow PN, Lobb EA, Analyzing the Process and Content of Genetic Counseling in Familial Breast Cancer Consultations. 2004. *J Genet Counsel*;13:403-24.

Chapter 13

1   Shiloh S, Saxe L. Perceptions of recurrence risks by genetic counselees. Psychol health 1989:45-61.

2   Gordon T, Edwards WS. *Making The Patient Your Partner*. Auburn House 1995 pp 213.

3   Dibben MR, Lean MEJ. Achieving compliance in chronic illness management: Illustrations of trust relationships between physicians and nutrition clinic patients. *Health Risk Soc.* 2003;5:241-58.

4   Frankel RM, Stein T, Krupat E, 2003. *Clinician-Patient Communication*, The Permanente Medical Group, Inc. (An update of Frankel and Stein. Getting the most out of the clinical encounter: the Four Habits Model. *Permanente J* 1999. Fall: 3(3);79-88.

5   Epstein RM, Alper BS, Quill TE, Communicating Evidence for Participatory Decision Making. *JAMA* 2004;291:2359-2366.

Chapter 14

1. PIAA Data Sharing Project. A Risk Management Review of Malpractice Claims: Combined Specialties. Physician Insurers Association Of America. 1985-2004. www.thepiaa.org

2 Levinson W. et al. Physician-patient communication: the relationship with malpractice claims among primary care physicians and surgeons. *JAMA* 1997; 277: 553-9 Also summarized in American Academy of Family Physicians web site www.aafp. org/970700ap/tips1.html).

3 Roter DL, Hall JA. How physician gender shapes the communication and evaluation of medical care. *Mayo Clin Proc* 2001: 76: 673-676.

4 Meeuwesen L, Van Der Staak C. Verbal analysis of doctor patient communication. *Soc Sci Med* 1991;32:1143-50.

5 Franks P, Clancy CM. Physician gender bias in clinical decision making: Screening for cancer in primary care. *Med Care* 1993;31:213-8.

6 Gray J. *Men Are from Mars, Women Are from Venus: a practical guide for improving communication and getting what you want in your relationships.* 1992. HarperCollins, 286 pp. ISBN:0060924160

7 Roter DL, Hall JA, Aoki Y, Physician Gender Effects in Medical Communication. A meta-analytical Review. *JAMA* August 14th 2002, Vol 288 No 6 pp 757-764.

Chapter 15

1 Singh AD, Paling JE. Informed consent: putting risks into perspective. *Surv Opthamol* 1997; 42: 83-86.

2 Lee DH, Paling JE, Blajchman MA. A new tool for communicating transfusion risk information. *Transfusion.* 1998;38:184-188.

3 Stallings SP, Paling JE. New tool for presenting risk in obstetrics and gynecology, *Obstet Gynecol* 2001;98:345-9.

4 Paling JE. Putting medical risks into perspective. In J.A.J. Barbara, J. Leikola, U. Rossi, editors, Risk perception and risk assessment in transfusion medicine: How to achieve a sound practice based on scientific truth. *Proceedings of the European School of Transfusion Medicine* Brussels 2003;99-112.

5 Kern DE, Thomas PA, Howard, DM, Bass EB. *Curriculum Development for Medical Education. A Six-Step Approach.* The Johns Hopkins University Press. 1998 ISBN 0-8018-5844-5.

Acknowledgments

So many people have given me input in researching and preparing this book that it is impossible to list everybody. However, I hope this general note will at least show my awareness of how they have influenced me on my journey. In particular I think of all the doctors and patients who have tested these tools and shared their experiences and frustrations about understanding risks.

A little extra time coupled with a wish to help are the key ingredients for superior doctor-patient communication. Exactly the same characteristics from reviewers have contributed greatly to this book. There are some who have given me so much time and help that they cannot pass unmentioned.

First and foremost Don Baumgart for his support and inspiration as we have developed the ideas (mainly his) for the series of illustrations for this book. His drawings constantly refreshed my own dedication to the project over its long gestation.

Next, I have been greatly helped by the many healthcare professionals who, despite being so busy, have given me their time and supportive suggestions. In particular: James Falconer Smith, Parker and Natalie Small, Kenneth Kellner, Sandra Leiblum, Mark Hochhauser, Adrian Edwards, Michelle Deschamps, Jim Rodrique, Samuel Sears, Allen Neims, William Chin, Adrianne Ingram, Don Price, Esme Nijland, Peter van de Weijer, Amie Stanley, Ann Marie Fenn, Dean Gabriel, Keith Stone, Chet Algood, Terry Stein, Robert Newman, Catherine Price, Mark Gold and Andrew Moore.

There are others who have given me so much detailed advice and support that I will always be indebted to them. Foremost in this category are Jonellen and Lou Heckler, and Bruce and Leslie Ingram. The depth of their contributions to this work were exceptional and I consider myself fortunate to have such generous friends.

Others gave me input on certain specialized aspects of the topic. Among these were Sean Paling, Valerie Moar, John Joplin, Karen Bradley and Beverly Clapp.

I also want to acknowledge research assistance from Catherine Bernstein of Physician Insurers Association of America, and Patricia Green of the Association of American Medical Colleges. Also Nancy Schaefer, Gloria London, Laurie Baker and Rick Lockwood and the staff of the Health Sciences Library at the University of Florida.

Lisa Baltozer, Shawna Mansfield, Jim Weems and Janice Phelps were the main advisors on the layout, cover design, and editing of the book. Ryan Rippel and Nicole Dudley contributed with additional graphics expertise throughout the project. In addition, I thank Dan Poynter and Greg Godek for guidance through the first steps into the maze of book production.

Finally I want to list some of those who have been special influences in my professional life, Bob Elliott, Stephen Covey, Ken Blanchard, Harvey MacKay, Stanley Hubbard, Jim Lazarus, David Machin, James McKay, Jean Gatz, Phillip Van Hooser, Don Blohowiak, Susan Friedmann, Jeff Tobe and Houston Wells. And last, but not least, Wendy, my wife of 25 years.

All these, and many others, helped me nurture the project. However, their suggestions were not always incorporated so, appropriately, the final responsibility for the book remains solely on the author's broad British back.

QUICK ORDER FORM

Satisfaction guaranteed

E-mail orders to: orders@riskcomm.com

Telephone Orders : Call 352 377 2142
Have your credit card ready

Postal Orders:
The Risk Communication Institute;
5822 N.W. 91 Blvd, Gainesville, Florida 32653

Please send the following books. I understand that I might return any of them for a full refund – for any reason, no questions asked.

(   ) copies of "Helping Patients Understand Risks".

See our website for additional information on:
Other books, Speaking/Seminars, Consulting.

Name:

Address:

City, State / Province, Post Code. Country.

Telephone:

E-mail:

Payment: Check, Credit card type.

Card number: Exp. date:

4537197

Made in the USA
Lexington, KY
04 February 2010